S0-AUR-062

IF IT RUNS IN YOUR FAMILY

COLORECTAL CANCER

REDUCING YOUR RISK

Bantam Books in the IF IT RUNS IN YOUR FAMILY series:

ALCOHOLISM
ARTHRITIS
BREAST CANCER
COLORECTAL CANCER
HEART DISEASE
OVARIAN AND UTERINE CANCER

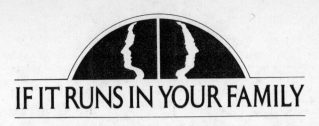

IF IT RUNS IN YOUR FAMILY

COLORECTAL CANCER

REDUCING YOUR RISK

Norman Sohn, M.D., and Scott Corngold

Foreword by William S. Haubrich, M.D., F.A.C.P.

Developed by The Philip Lief Group, Inc.

BANTAM BOOKS
NEW YORK · TORONTO · LONDON · SYDNEY · AUCKLAND

This book is not intended as a substitute for the medical advice of physicians. The reader should regularly consult a physician in matters relating to his or her health and particularly with respect to any symptoms that may require diagnosis or medical attention. Readers should also speak with their own doctors about their own individual needs before starting any diet or fitness program. Consulting one's personal physician about diet and exercise is especially important if the reader is on any medication or is already under medical care for any illness.

IF IT RUNS IN YOUR FAMILY: COLORECTAL CANCER
A Bantam Book/May 1992

All rights reserved.
Copyright © 1992 by The Philip Lief Group, Inc.
Cover art copyright © 1992 by Eye Tooth Design, Inc.
No part of this book may be reproduced or transmitted
in any form or by any means, electronic or mechanical,
including photocopying, recording, or by any information
storage and retrieval system, without permission in writing from
the publisher.
For information address: Bantam Books.

Library of Congress Cataloging-in-Publication Data

Sohn, Norman.
    If it runs in your family—colorectal cancer : reducing your risk
/ Norman Sohn and Scott Corngold ; foreword by William S. Haubrich ;
developed by the Philip Lief Group, Inc.
        p.   cm.
    Includes bibliographical references and index.
    ISBN 0-553-35173-7
    1. Colon (Anatomy)—Cancer—Popular works.   2. rectum—Cancer—

Popular works.   I. Corngold, Scott.   II. Philip Lief Group.
III. Title.
RC280.C6S64   1992
616.99'4347—dc20   91-40424
                                                                    CIP

Published simultaneously in the United States and Canada

Bantam Books are published by Bantam Books, a division of Bantam Doubleday
Dell Publishing Group, Inc. Its trademark, consisting of the words "Bantam Books"
and the portrayal of a rooster, is Registered in U.S. Patent and Trademark Office
and in other countries. Marca Registrada. Bantam Books, 666 Fifth Avenue, New
York, New York 10103.

PRINTED IN THE UNITED STATES OF AMERICA
OPM   0   9   8   7   6   5   4   3   2   1

Acknowledgments

We would like to thank the following individuals for their editorial guidance and assistance: Cathy Hemming, Jamie Rothstein, Alan Mahony, Lisa Schwartzburg, Lee Ann Chearneyi, Julia Banks, and Becky Cabaza. Our appreciation also to Dr. William Haubrich for his review of the manuscript.

Contents

Foreword

The message is all here: the bane and the boon. The bane is the pervasive threat of colorectal cancer; the boon is that we can take measures to lessen the threat. The authors of *If It Runs in Your Family: Colorectal Cancer* have done a creditable job of explaining what we must face when contending with the most prevalent of cancers afflicting the gastrointestinal tract. If to be forewarned is to be forearmed, here is the up-to-date information individuals need in order to deal with this potentially deadly foe.

In chapter 1 the problem is put into proper perspective. Yes, we are all at risk, but for some of us the risk may be greater than for others. No, we cannot entirely eliminate the risk, but there are ways to reduce it.

Risk factors emerging from our own individual health histories are detailed in chapter 2. These factors include circumstances that may potentially be precursors of colon cancer and that mandate particular attention, such as familial polyposis.

Chapter 3 tells what is known and what is being learned about the role of heredity in predicting our risk of colorectal cancer. One of my professors in medical school once said, "The secret to a long and healthy life is to pick the right ancestors." The truth—and the irony—of this pronouncement is increasingly evident. Neither I nor anyone I know has had the privilege of assembling ancestors of choice, but the benefits of knowing your family medical history are vast.

In chapter 4 the authors venture into less certain and more controversial territory when they explain the presumed role of environmental factors, including diet, and their impact on the risk of developing colorectal cancer. The advice given, in the light of growing current knowledge, is sensible.

The next three chapters give a well-focused picture of the symptoms that can betray the presence of cancer in the colon or rectum, the procedures doctors use to seek out and identify suspected growths in the bowel, and the means by which discovered lesions can be effectively treated. The book concludes with a justifiably optimistic look at the benefits ongoing advances may provide in the near future.

I heartily agree with the authors' principal theme: that lessening the risk of colorectal cancer demands a close and well-informed partnership between patient and physician. This book can serve as a sound step in helping to establish and further that partnership.

WILLIAM S. HAUBRICH, M.D., F.A.C.P.,
Senior Consultant in Gastroenterology, Emeritus,
Scripps Clinic and Research Foundation
Clinical Professor of Medicine,
University of California, San Diego

IF IT RUNS IN YOUR FAMILY

COLORECTAL CANCER

REDUCING YOUR RISK

1

Learning the Facts, Confronting the Fear

It is a disease that strikes one in twenty Americans. It is the second most common cancer in the United States and the second leading cause of cancer death, after lung cancer. In 1992, almost 160,000 people will be diagnosed for the disease; more than 60,000 will die from it. Yet these statistics could be different if more Americans knew the right steps to take.

We're talking about colorectal cancer. It's something, admittedly, no one much likes to talk about or think about. It's also both highly preventable and highly curable, only the rates aren't dropping the way they should be . . . largely because no one likes to talk about it or think about it.

When Ronald Reagan's colorectal cancer was diagnosed in 1985, we could hardly *help* talking about it or thinking about it. Graphic diagrams of the president's diseased colon were regularly beamed onto our television screens and splashed across the pages of our newspapers. Interview after interview with oncologists, proctologists, and gastroenterologists were followed by commentaries from pundits of the press: Were the president's doctors treating the disease correctly? What was his prognosis? Why wasn't the cancer found earlier? What are *your* chances of getting it?

Reagan's battle with colorectal cancer did a lot to bring the disease to the public's attention and to educate us about its prevalence and its dangers. But seven years have passed and we have another president, and other diseases, on our minds. It's been very easy to forget what we learned about colorectal cancer—and to forget our promises to ourselves to learn more.

No one much likes talking or thinking about cancer at all. But there's something about disorders and malignant growths in the colon and rectum that makes colorectal cancer a subject we'd go to even greater lengths to avoid. Let's face it, when you're talking about colorectal cancer, you're talking about bowel habits. You're talking about bloody stools and flatulence and diarrhea and constipation. You're talking about insidious growths and about exams using intimidating tools that probe deep into the most private and tender parts of our bodies. No wonder it ranks close to the bottom of our list of preferred conversation topics.

We're being blunt here right off the bat, because it's so crucial to remove the stigma from this subject and get past our reluctance to deal with the sometimes discomforting information about cancer of the large bowel. You may never feel completely comfortable talking about this disease, but it is important to be knowledgeable about the facts: how colorectal cancer develops, how its genetic component places some families at higher risk, and how you can take steps to reduce your likelihood of getting the disease. And that requires a willingness to explore some sensitive material and to discuss it with your physician—and with your family.

Getting the Facts Straight

Here are some of the basic facts about colorectal cancer:

• Colorectal cancer occurs most frequently in the United States, Europe, Australia, and New Zealand. It is far rarer in Japan and most of the developing nations. In the United States, colorectal cancer rates are highest in the Northeast and in large urban areas and are lowest in the South and Southwest. The disease is also less common among Seventh-Day Adventists and other vegetarians.

• Colorectal cancer is not a rare disease; it is the second most common form of cancer in the United States. In this country in this year alone, it is estimated there will be 157,500 new cases of colorectal cancer (compared with 160,000 new cases of lung cancer); 111,500 will be cancers of the colon and 46,000 will be malignancies of the rectum.

• The incidence of colorectal cancer in the United States rose by almost 10 percent from 1973 to 1985. Part of the increase is due to the rise in the number of elderly, who are more likely to develop the disease.

• Men and women develop the disease in largely equal numbers. Among men it is the third most common form of cancer (lung cancer is first, prostate cancer is second), while among women it is the second most common form (breast cancer is first).

• For Americans over the age of twenty, colorectal cancer is slightly more prevalent among whites than blacks. But for reasons that aren't clear, the mortality rates are higher among blacks. The explanation may have to do with the fact that larger numbers of African-Americans lack access to proper medical care.

• One-quarter of all people with colorectal cancer have a clear family history of the disease. People with one or more close relatives who have had colorectal cancer are two to four times more likely to develop the disease—a 10 to 15 percent chance over the course of a lifetime—than people in families not afflicted with the disease.

•   This year, an estimated 61,000 people in the United States will die from colorectal cancer, making it the second leading cause of cancer death in this country. It is the second leading cause of cancer death among men (after lung cancer) and the third leading cause of cancer death among women (after breast and lung cancer).

•   Colorectal cancer is not always fatal. The current five-year survival rate among colorectal cancer patients in the United States is around 53 percent, up from 40 percent in the 1950s. The rate is expected to rise further by the end of the century.

•   The survival rate could be much higher. If detected in its early stage, colorectal cancer is curable in more than 90 percent of cases. That cure rate is higher than for virtually every other form of cancer. On the other hand, fewer than one-third of those with advanced cancer of the large bowel will survive beyond five years.

•   Readily available, relatively inexpensive diagnostic exams may be able to detect early-stage malignancies in the colon and rectum more than 90 percent of the time. Yet surveys indicate that fewer than half of all Americans at high risk of developing colorectal cancer have ever undergone the recommended examinations.

Who Should Read This Book

This book is for those who don't want to accept the kind of ignorance and fear that keeps so many people from dealing effectively with a disease like cancer. It is for people who believe they, or someone they care about, may be at risk of developing colorectal cancer . . . and who want to do something about it. Perhaps several of your family members have had the disease. Or your doctor may have determined that you have a condition that makes you more vulnerable to the disease. Maybe you recently turned forty, and have heard that colorectal cancer is more prevalent once you've reached middle age. Or maybe you're concerned about all that talk about fat and fiber and worry that you're eating too much of one and not enough of the other. And you might be wondering whether a minor physical complaint you've been experiencing recently might be indicating something serious. We'll be discussing all this and more.

No one, as far as we know, is entirely free of all risk of developing colorectal cancer. But several factors can increase your likelihood of getting it. The key risk factors for colorectal cancer fall into three general categories, and we will be reviewing each of them in detail. These are

- Personal health background.
- Family background.
- Environmental influences.

Most of the time, a combination of several factors affects colorectal cancer development. This book will help you learn which ones affect you, which ones don't, and which ones you can do something about.

You'll learn how to determine patterns in your family history that may mean you—or your children—are at risk of colorectal cancer. We'll discuss which features in your health background, your diet, and your lifestyle practices also place you at higher risk. And you'll find out how to begin to take the proper steps to reduce that risk significantly.

In the process, you'll be neutralizing that other crucial, yet overlooked, factor that places so many Americans at risk: ignorance—ignorance about colorectal cancer, about what you may be doing to increase your chances of getting it, and about what you *could* be doing to prevent it.

As you read this book, you may confirm, if you weren't sure

already, that you or someone you love is indeed at risk of colorectal cancer. That shouldn't make you panic. Instead, it should motivate you and encourage you to make changes that may save your life. Armed with the right information, you can turn "at risk" to "in control"—of your own health and future as well as the health and future of your family.

2

Your Health Background

SELF-TEST

Many aspects of your personal health history need to be considered in evaluating your level of risk for contracting colorectal cancer. To compile an accurate record of relevant information, answer the following questions.

		Score
1.	Are you forty or older?	_____
2.	Have you ever had a polyp removed from your large bowel?	_____
3.	Do you have ulcerative colitis?	
	If so: Has it been active for ten years or more?	_____
	Did it first develop during childhood?	_____
	Does it involve most of your colon or your entire colon?	_____

4. Do you have Crohn's disease?   _____
5. Have you ever had a cancerous tumor
    removed from the large intestine?   _____
6. *(For women)* Do you have a history of
    breast, ovarian, cervical, or uterine cancer?   _____
7. Have you had radiation treatment in the
    pelvic area?   _____
8. Have you had surgery to remove your gall-
    bladder?   _____
9. Have you had surgery to implant a ureter?   _____

Now read on to find out exactly how these factors may increase your likelihood of developing colorectal cancer.

Anatomy of the Large Intestine

To understand how colorectal cancer develops and how aspects
of your health background may make you vulnerable to the
disease, you need to have a basic idea of how the large intestine
works. So let's begin with a brief anatomy lesson.

The colon and rectum together make up the large intestine,
also called the large bowel. This is the lower portion of the
human digestive tract. By the time the food we've eaten reaches
the large bowel, it has already been digested in the small intestine,
also called the small bowel. There, nutrients in the food have
been broken down into chemical units small enough to pass
through the intestinal wall and into the bloodstream and *lymphatic system* to be sent through the entire body. The remaining
undigested food, water, and waste flows in semiliquid form from
the *ileum,* the last division of the small intestine located in the
lower right-hand side of the abdomen, into the *cecum,* a pouch-
like chamber that is the first portion of the large bowel (Figure
1).

The colon acts as a reservoir for waste material as the body

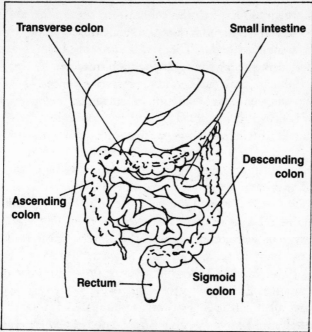

Figure 1. Diagram of the large intestine.

completes the digestion process. In the colon, most of the water, as well as vital body salts such as sodium and potassium, is extracted from the unwanted remains of the meal (forwarded from the small bowel) and is absorbed into the cells lining the intestine. The water and salts will soon go elsewhere in the body. The waste, meanwhile, which has become semisolid stool after the absorption of the water, remains in the colon, where many different bacteria that are naturally contained there break down the remaining carbohydrates and proteins and convert still-undigested food components into several kinds of vitamins.

This fecal material is moved through the entire length of the large intestine, as it was through the small intestine, by regular involuntary muscular contractions. The bowel walls contain cells that produce mucus to lubricate and protect the intestinal surface as the waste material continues on its way.

The large intestine is usually about 4 to 6 feet long and 1 to 3 inches in diameter, wider than the small intestine. It is divided into six areas. The cecum, the first portion of the large bowel, is located in the lower right-hand section of the abdomen, with the appendix, a small, narrow tube, extending from it. The colon heads up the right side of the abdomen toward the liver. This portion is called the *ascending colon*. It then crosses the abdomen, as the *transverse colon,* under the stomach toward the spleen. There it becomes the *descending colon,* going down the abdomen's left side to the pelvis, curving at the S-shaped *sigmoid colon.* The *rectum* is the last portion of the large bowel, a 4- to 6-inch-long section, where the feces are stored until eliminated through the anus as a bowel movement.

The stay of undigested food in the large intestine is brief, taking only about 12 to 14 hours to pass through the entire snaking passageway. Cancer of the large bowel, of course, remains far longer. It actually grows surprisingly slowly: The doubling time of a cancer cell averages about two years, while a normal cell in the large intestine is replicated in about five days. Colorectal cancer can take ten, twenty, or more years to develop, because a number of mutational events are necessary for a line of cells in the bowel to start producing out of control.

How Colorectal Cancer Develops

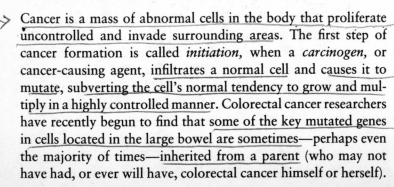

Cancer is a mass of abnormal cells in the body that proliferate uncontrolled and invade surrounding areas. The first step of cancer formation is called *initiation,* when a *carcinogen,* or cancer-causing agent, infiltrates a normal cell and causes it to mutate, subverting the cell's normal tendency to grow and multiply in a highly controlled manner. Colorectal cancer researchers have recently begun to find that some of the key mutated genes in cells located in the large bowel are sometimes—perhaps even the majority of times—inherited from a parent (who may not have had, or ever will have, colorectal cancer himself or herself).

The second step of cancer development is *promotion,* when substances that are not carcinogenic themselves aid the activity and development of *potentially* malignant cells.

In the large intestine, the first sign of irregular activity is *dysplasia,* an excess accumulation of cells along the bowel wall, or the presence of *benign polyps,* from which perhaps 90 percent of all colorectal cancers grow. (Colorectal cancer can develop even without the presence of polyps in the large bowel, but it's about five times more likely that polyps will either precede or be present at the same time as a malignancy.) Polyps are small, usually harmless tumors, or tissue masses, that generally grow on the inner surface of the intestine. The size can vary from less than two-tenths of an inch to more than 2 inches in diameter, and there are several different types. The least serious is called a hyperplastic polyp, a tiny lesion made up of a rearranged mass of excess cells lining the bowel that is likely to stay small and is not considered to be part of the cancer-development process. About 25 percent of all polyps found, and most of those found in the rectum, are this type of growth.

Other polyps, called *adenomas,* are lesions that project into the bowel channel (lumen) from a stalklike connection to the bowel surface. They, too, tend to be—and to remain—small and the great majority are unlikely ever to develop into cancer. Adenomas often look like a grape and have a relatively smooth surface.

Still, an adenoma may continue to grow and cancer cells may form within it. In general, the larger the polyp, the greater chance there is for cancer to be present. Those larger than three-quarters of an inch are especially ominous, but most adenomas found in the intestine are much smaller. The three most common adenomas are tubular, villous, and intermediate (or tubulovillous). Tubular adenomas are usually distributed throughout the large intestine, whereas villous adenomas, which have irregular, fingerlike projections, are more frequently found in the rectum. (This is only a generalization, however. The cancerous tumor found in Ronald Reagan, for example, was a villous adenoma located in the cecum, all the way at the other end of his bowel.) Tubular adenomas, believed to occur in up to 15 percent of the adult population, are four times more common than the villous type and are most often smaller. About 5 percent of these growths will become malignant. Villous adenomas, perhaps because of their tendency to be larger, are eight to ten times more likely to be cancerous. Intermediate polyps are somewhat more common than villous growths but are less frequently malignant.

Polyps are more likely to grow in the rectum and sigmoid colon than in the other sections of the large intestine, which is good in that those are the parts most accessible in examinations. But, for unknown reasons, there has been a progressive increase of cancer located higher in the colon, toward the right-hand side, in the ascending colon and cecum. Fortunately, screening exams have progressed to a state where this portion of the large bowel can also be thoroughly checked.

In its earliest stage, colorectal cancer is usually very superficial—and very curable—involving only the lining of the intestine, without invading, or only beginning to penetrate, the bowel wall or muscle layer. In its more advanced stages, however, the cancer will erode through the entire wall and involve the lymph nodes (which filter bacteria and abnormal matter from the watery fluid between cells) within the abdomen. If the cancer spreads to the lymphatic system, malignant cells may be ferried throughout the body where they can lodge, multiply, and form new tumors, a process called *metastasis*. And in its most serious stage, when the prognosis is particularly poor, the cancer spreads into the liver or other nearby organs.

But that only happens when the cancer hasn't been caught in its early stages. And it certainly *can* be caught early. In the first place, compared with other malignant tumors, tumors in the colon and rectum grow rather slowly. (The doubling time of the tumor—a somewhat objective measure of the rate of growth, defined as the time necessary for the tumor to double its volume—for primary colorectal cancer

$$90 \text{ wks} = 1 \text{ yr, } 9 \text{ mos.}$$
$$\begin{array}{r} -52 \\ \hline 38 \end{array}$$

is ninety weeks. For lung cancer the average doubling time is twelve to twenty-one weeks, breast cancer fourteen weeks, and lymphoma four weeks.) Plus, unlike many other cancers, colorectal cancer is usually detectable in its initial, highly curable stages—if the recommended screening procedures are followed. You can even spot and take care of trouble before any cancer develops. That's why it's so crucial to learn if you, or someone you know, is at a high risk of developing the disease. Then you can be on guard for, and treat, the most vestigial signs of the evolving disease and avoid practices that may provoke or encourage cancer growth.

The risk factors for colorectal cancer can be divided into three broad categories—health background, hereditary background, and environmental contributions. Let's begin by discussing the influences in your health background that may make you especially vulnerable to colorectal cancer.

Health Background Risk Factors

Age

A major reason colorectal cancer rates are rising in the United States is because people are living longer. Cancer of the large bowel is a disease of age. Remember that cancer takes decades to develop in the large bowel; the older you are, the more time malignant cells in the colon and rectum have to develop and multiply. Consequently, the likelihood of developing colorectal cancer increases with advancing age.

Although colorectal cancer is sometimes found in children, only about 1 percent of all malignant tumors of the large bowel are found in people under age thirty. More than 90 percent appear in people fifty years or older. But the incidence begins increasing steadily from age forty (earlier among those with a family history of colorectal cancer) up to the eighth decade and peaking at around age seventy-five. To give you an idea of how your risk for colorectal cancer increases with age, Table 1 lists 1988 statistics from the National Cancer Institute showing the rates for the disease among Americans.

Table 1. Annual Incidence of Colorectal Cancer (per 100,000)

Age	White Males	Black Males	White Females	Black Females
40–49	20.3	26.8	19.8	23.5
50–59	83.4	86.0	67.7	73.9
60–69	230.1	209.0	155.4	168.7
70–79	449.5	392.3	312.8	305.5

The critical fact here is that you are considered to be at moderate risk of developing colorectal cancer once you reach age forty and at high risk once you turn fifty, regardless of your health profile or family background. Medical experts uniformly agree that *all* people over forty years old should begin to be screened regularly for the disease, even if nothing in their lifestyle, diet, health, and family history shows any warning signs for cancer.

Polyps

If your doctor finds that you have a polyp, you won't have it for long. Polyps of any size in the large intestine, whether or not they are cancerous, are almost always removed once they're detected. But although the growth itself is gone, you nevertheless now have a history of polyps, and that places you at considerably higher risk of developing colorectal cancer. And if you have even the smallest, most benign kind of adenoma and it *hasn't* been found, because you haven't undergone regular or sufficiently thorough screening examinations, then that tumor remains embedded in your bowel wall where it can grow and turn cancerous.

About 10 to 15 percent of all Americans—and especially older people—develop polyps in the colon and rectum. As we've discussed, most of these growths are very small and entirely harmless. Nevertheless, a polyp of any size should be removed. That's because, although they're rarely cancerous, they can grow and eventually develop a malignancy. And even if there is no threat of cancer, large polyps can cause you some major digestive troubles. Furthermore, a doctor cannot know for certain whether a polyp actually is cancerous without performing a *biopsy,* and oftentimes, the procedure to remove a polyp is as simple as the procedure to obtain the tissue necessary for a biopsy in the first place. Most polyps, except for the largest ones, can be removed without surgery, often during the very screening exam when they are first detected.

It's not always necessary, however (particularly with hyperplastic polyps, which are invariably benign), to have them removed right after detection. Frequently, when a polyp found during a routine screening is not believed to be cancerous, a doctor may postpone its removal until a more thorough examination for other polyps can be performed. President Reagan's cancer, in fact, was discovered in July 1985, when his entire colon was inspected during the removal of a one-seventh–inch polyp that had been found four months earlier. While it is not always advisable (even if you're as busy as a world leader) to postpone removal of a polyp *(polypectomy)* that long—and, indeed, Reagan's physicians received strong criticism from some medical circles—that relatively short amount of time probably doesn't make much difference, as long as a complete examination for other growths is made. The wisest course, nevertheless, is usually not to take chances and to schedule a polypectomy relatively soon after the tumor is discovered.

Even if they're not discovered and removed, polyps rarely grow larger than one-fifth of an inch, and within that size they are highly likely to remain benign. Only 2.5 to 5 percent of all polyps ever eventually become malignant. Remember, though, that the larger the polyp, the greater the possibility that it will be cancerous. Recent findings show that generally:

- 1 percent of polyps two-fifths of an inch in diameter or smaller are found to contain cancer.
- 10 to 20 percent of polyps two-fifths to three-quarters of an inch in diameter contain cancer.
- Approximately 50 percent of polyps larger than 1⅕ inches in diameter contain cancer.
- Close to 100 percent of polyps larger than 2 inches in diameter contain cancer.

It is important to keep in mind that even the smallest polyp is detectable in a sufficiently thorough screening and even the biggest polyp probably doesn't start out cancerous.

An adenoma as large as 2 inches has probably been growing in the large intestine for years. And in all that time, as it was growing and becoming malignant it could have been detected— quite possibly when it was still benign.

When the Polyp Is Removed. If you've been diligent, received regular colorectal exams, and caught a polyp in its early, benign stage, you're still not quite out of the woods. The fact that you have had a polyp should fortify your resolve to continue being careful. Because it means that you are significantly more likely than the average person to develop another polyp in the future— or to have more polyps currently growing farther up in the colon. And, logically, the more polyps you have growing, the greater the chance that cancer will develop.

If one polyp is found, there's a 40 to 50 percent chance you have another one growing elsewhere in the bowel. That's why it is very wise to have the entire colon examined after the discovery of any polyp, even one located in the rectum. When Reagan's first two hyperplastic polyps were found, in 1984 and in March 1985, he did not undergo a complete colorectal screening, and when the second polyp was finally removed, doctors found a cancerous 2-inch villous adenoma that had been growing all along.

There's also about a 30 percent chance you'll develop another polyp sometime in the future, with the risk of recurrence increasing three to five years after discovery of the previous one. It's somewhat more likely to happen if you have had multiple villous polyps, but even a singular tubular polyp in your past means that you run a higher risk of developing more polyps in the future. The bottom line is that *once you've had a polyp, it's even more important to continue undergoing regular colorectal screening.*

Inflammatory Bowel Disease

Two million Americans suffer from *ulcerative colitis,* or *Crohn's disease.* These are serious, long-term disorders, often referred to as inflammatory bowel disease, that can be highly disruptive of your daily life. Colitis can also greatly increase your chances—up to thirty times—of developing colorectal cancer.

Ulcerative colitis is the chronic inflammation of either part of or the entire large intestine. Tiny breaks develop on the colon's inner surface causing tissue to die and patches of the lining to slough off. This can leave substantial areas ulcerated and unable to perform the colon's job of absorbing water and minerals from digested food. And when the disease is in an active phase, it can also leave you feeling pretty lousy, suffering from bloody diarrhea, fever, abdominal pain and cramps, weight loss, and anemia. Like stomach ulcers, it can even cause a perforation of the organ.

Ulcerative colitis most commonly first strikes anywhere from the teens through the early thirties—75 percent of colitis cases begin before age forty. The disease may remain your entire life, with long periods of inactivity followed by flare-ups.

It is thought that in perhaps 10 percent of the cases, colitis involves a hereditary factor, and more than one member of individual families can be affected. The exact cause of the disease is unknown, and doctors are not in complete agreement about whether stress and other emotional factors may predispose certain people or exacerbate the condition. (*Irritable bowel syndrome,* which shares many symptoms with colitis, but is, nevertheless, an entirely different condition unassociated with a higher cancer risk, is decidedly stress related.)

The food you eat may also be related, and although some doctors question its effectiveness, treatment for colitis often involves a special diet. The specifics depend on the severity of the condition but are most likely to entail limiting consumption of dairy products, nuts and seeds, roughage, and/or high-gluten grains like wheat and rye. Medication is frequently prescribed— most commonly steroids and antibiotics but mild sedatives or antispasmodic drugs may also be given—and rest is recommended as well. Your doctor will provide a balanced program gauged for the specific characteristics of your condition.

With care, most colitis patients live perfectly normal lives, and many may need no special treatment at all. No cure, however, is known, except for surgery to remove the colon, and that is performed only in the most serious, life-threatening cases that involve only very few colitis sufferers.

About one in one hundred people with colorectal cancer have a background of ulcerative colitis. In general, colitis patients have a three times greater chance of developing colorectal cancer than the general population. So if you have colitis, you should consider yourself at high risk. But although in the broadest terms a person with colitis may have a 15 percent chance of eventually getting cancer, the risk can vary greatly depending on severity and duration of the disease. People who have only transient episodes of *proctitis* (inflammation of the rectum alone) do not seem to have a higher incidence of cancer at all. The risk is greater, however, if:

- Your colitis has been active for more than ten years.
- Your colitis involves most of, or the entire, colon.
- You developed colitis at an early age.

The longer you have had colitis and the more serious the condition, the likelier your chances are of developing cancer. In fact, your risk is said to increase by 20 percent for each decade after diagnosis. People affected with active colitis involving most of the large intestine for more than twenty years are especially predisposed, and some researchers have estimated that those who have had a severe colitis condition for more than thirty years may have a greater than 35 percent chance of developing colorectal cancer. The likelihood is increased further if you have suffered from colitis since childhood, although this is not as important a factor as the first two.

If you have Crohn's disease, an inflammatory condition similar to ulcerative colitis that occurs most often in the ileum and parts of the colon, you also have an increased risk of colorectal cancer. It is not, however, nearly as frequently associated with cancer as ulcerative colitis.

Although some severe cases of colitis (and Crohn's disease) are treated with abdominal surgery, the only time surgery is considered as a preventive measure against cancer would be in the uncommon case when the condition is accompanied by severe dysplasia, a strong indication that cancer cell growth may be imminent.

Nevertheless, people with chronic inflammatory bowel disease can practice cancer prevention—and practice it effectively—by following the prescribed medication and diet regimen that keeps the colitis under control and by dealing appropriately with the environmental factors that decrease, or further increase, their risk. Even more crucial, along with other high-risk groups, people with colitis should undergo cancer screening more often, and starting at an earlier age, than the general population. This includes, ideally, an annual *endoscopic* examination of the colon interior (we'll be discussing this later), which, as well as checking for dysplasia, developing polyps, and cancer, is also necessary to monitor the progress of the colitis itself.

Previous Colorectal Cancer and Other Conditions

Among the key groups of people most likely to develop cancer of the large bowel are those who have had it in the past. People who have undergone treatment for colorectal cancer don't merely run the risk of that cancer recurring. About 5 to 10 percent of them eventually develop a second cancerous tumor in the large bowel, making them three times more likely than the general population to have a brand new episode of colorectal cancer.

People who have a history of other kinds of cancer are also at greater risk of developing colorectal cancer. Women with breast or ovarian cancer are about one and a half times more likely than the general population to have a malignancy in the large intestine concurrently or to develop one in the future. That's because many women with a history of those cancers possess the hereditary trait of "family cancer syndrome" (which we'll discuss in the next chapter).

One study of women with breast cancer who also have a family history of gastrointestinal cancer showed them to be at four and a half times greater risk than the general population of developing colorectal cancer, a significantly higher risk increase than women with a similar family background but without a personal history of breast cancer. Because of this connection, most doctors strongly recommend that you be screened for colorectal cancer if you learn you have breast, ovarian, or uterine cancer (and vice versa), and that you be regularly screened thereafter.

Sometimes it's the treatment of the disease, rather than the condition itself, that places a person at higher risk. Radiation treatment of the pelvic area, performed on people who have cervical, uterine, or bladder cancer, seems to increase the chances of colorectal cancer development. Researchers aren't sure why, but theorize that the radiation may introduce a particularly high number of carcinogens into the large intestine.

If you've had your gallbladder removed or have had a ureter implanted to carry urine from the kidney, you are also at higher risk for colorectal cancer. The reason for this is also unclear, but the best guess is that secretions in the abdomen caused by these operations may contain carcinogens or other cancer-promoting compounds.

Questions and Answers

Q: I'm in my early twenties. If colorectal cancer doesn't usually strike until much later in life, why should I worry about it now?

A: Although it's true that the vast majority of colorectal cancer patients are over forty, younger people, even in their early teens, can develop it as well, particularly those in some families with a genetic susceptibility to the disease. But even though the chances are highly unlikely that you will get colorectal cancer this early in life, it still pays to be aware. Cancer, after all, doesn't just happen overnight. It takes years to grow, and it's often caused—and avoided—by the habits of a lifetime. Now is exactly the time to learn about cancer of the large bowel and especially to learn about what you are doing that might be placing you at higher risk—and what you can do to reduce your chances of ever developing it.

Q: Can a person ever have so many repeated episodes of polyps that some kind of surgical procedure is recommended?

A: Some people affected by a relatively rare inherited condition called familial polyposis, which we'll discuss in the next chapter, develop literally hundreds of polyps in the colon or rectum, often well before adulthood. For those individuals, it's usually recommended that the colon, or the colon and rectum, be removed when the condition is first observed, to prevent the almost inevitable development of a cancerous tumor. In most cases, however, people affected by polyps have no more than a few. Since the growths are rarely cancerous and because the procedure to remove them is usually a simple one, it's better to take care of each polyp as it appears rather than go to any surgical extremes.

Q: I have had ulcerative colitis for almost twenty years, since age seventeen. It's a minor condition, mostly affecting only the rectum, and I haven't had to take any medication for it for years. Do I still run a higher risk of developing colorectal cancer?

A: There's no exact way to quantify your risk for colorectal cancer. Because you have had the condition for so long, you are probably somewhat more vulnerable than the general population, especially because dysplasia, believed to be an early precursor of malignancy, can be seen in even mild cases of proctitis. But the mildness of the condition puts you at much lower risk than those who have had active colitis affecting most of the bowel for so long a period of time.

Nevertheless, even though you have not needed medication for some time, you should still be getting endoscopic exams regularly to monitor the progress of the disease. Those tests should reveal any exacerbation of your condition and also spot any benign adenomas or cancerous tumors that may be developing. Discuss this with your doctor if you haven't been to see him or her recently.

Q: I don't understand how someone who's had colorectal cancer can get it again. Once you've had it, isn't the large intestine removed?

A: Colorectal cancer is often treated (as we'll see in chapter 7) by surgery, but it's a common misunderstanding that the discovery of this cancer automatically means removal of the entire large bowel and the necessity of a *colostomy* (a surgical procedure in which the diseased section of the intestinal tract is removed and an opening called a stoma is made in the abdominal wall). More often than not, only the part of the bowel that is affected (along with a portion on both sides, just to make sure) is removed, the remaining sections surgically reattached with no need at all for a colostomy. That leaves a good portion of the large intestine intact, where there is a chance that another malignancy may grow in the future.

Q: If radiation can promote the development of colorectal cancer, should I be concerned about X rays?

A: The amount of radiation to which your body is exposed in radiation treatment of the pelvis for diseases like cervical, uterine, or bladder cancer is far, far more intense than radiation from a simple X ray. You do get exposed to a small amount, but doctors are acutely aware of the dangers of radiation, and most are quite prudent about their X-ray recommendations. And the risk from an occasional sensibly recommended and carefully performed X ray is certainly offset by the benefits.

3

Your Family Background

Just how much does your family history influence your risk of developing colorectal cancer? For a long time, the connection between heredity and colorectal cancer was underestimated, considered tenuous at best. Cancer of the large bowel seemed to result primarily from the inevitable aging process, helped along by several suspected, yet not clearly identified, environmental factors. With few exceptions, when members of a single family— even across several generations—developed the disease, coincidence or shared lifestyles appeared to be as likely explanations as any possible genetic link.

Nevertheless, many researchers had a nagging suspicion that heredity played a bigger role than had been assumed. They pointed to certain syndromes well known to be inherited, like *familial polyposis* (a condition causing the development of multiple polyps), which clearly placed some families at very high risk of colorectal cancer. Could there be other genetic susceptibilities that, perhaps less inevitably but still decidedly, predisposed some families to the disease as well? Could a tendency to develop colorectal cancer be passed from generation to generation?

Genetic Theory in Brief

A human cell contains two sets of twenty-three *chromosomes*. We inherit one set from both parents. These chromosomes are made up of long, spiraling chains of deoxyribonucleic acid (better known as *DNA*), which hold the *genome*, our complete set of about 100,000 *genes*. Genes direct the cell to produce the proteins that carry out all the functions of life and determine our very individual physical characteristics, from the color of our eyes, to if (and when) we'll go bald, to the possible presence of certain diseases and physical problems we may either experience from birth or develop somewhere down the line. Some of these malfunctions are caused by mutations in the genes, which may have occurred due to some environmental factor or may have simply been passed on that way from one or both of our parents. Tay-Sachs disease and sickle-cell anemia are two of the more familiar inherited genetic disorders. The genes causing them have been identified, so that doctors can determine prenatally, through amniocentesis, whether a child will have either condition.

The rules of genetic inheritance were first deciphered in the nineteenth century by Gregor Mendel. A monk who traced and recorded information about dominant and recessive genetic transmission, Mendel used a monastery garden as his laboratory by studying the traits of pea plants. He discovered that by cross-pollinating these plants in a controlled fashion, he could determine the attributes of a seedling plant based on the traits of the parent plants.

Because he kept exhaustive records, Mendel was able to ascertain that some traits would be passed on to the offspring if just one parent possessed them (dominant traits) and some would only be inherited if both parents carried them (recessive traits). He also determined the basic mathematical rule for the likelihood of an offspring to receive dominant and recessive traits. Although these rules don't apply to all cases of inheritance, they form the basis for the science of genetics and are fundamental to our understanding of the genetics of colorectal cancer.

Here is a brief example to illustrate these rules. Remember that organisms, from pea plants to humans, receive one-half of their genes from each parent. For this illustration, we'll assume that a single gene pair controls the trait, although in many cases—including, geneticists believe, colorectal cancer—the expression, or physical manifestation, of a trait depends on the interplay and contribution of multiple gene pairs. For our example, we'll use eye color, and to simplify, we'll limit the discussion to brown eyes and blue eyes.

Brown eyes is a dominant trait, meaning the allele (one member of the "pair" that makes up the gene) for brown eyes will be expressed whenever it is present. So a person who receives this allele from one parent will, indeed, have brown eyes, even if the allele he or she receives from the other parent is an allele for blue eyes. Blue eyes, on the other hand, is a recessive trait. A person would have to carry two blue-eyed alleles in order actually to have blue eyes.

What happens when a brown-eyed person and a blue-eyed person have a child? Let's take the case where both parents carry pure strains of the trait, meaning that the brown-eyed parent possesses two brown-eyed alleles (we'll designate B, using the upper case, to represent the dominant form of the eye-color gene), and the blue-eyed parent possesses two recessive alleles (which we'll designate as b). These individuals are referred to as being homozygous because they each possess only one form of the eye-color gene.

Because each parent will pass along one of his or her two eye-color genes, there are four possible gene pairs that each offspring could receive. In this case, the brown-eyed parent has only a dominant brown-eyed allele to pass on to his or her offspring; likewise, the blue-eyed parent can only pass on a recessive, blue-eyed allele. Thus the eye-color gene pair in each offspring will be the same for each of the four possible pairings:

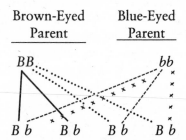

Brown-Eyed   Blue-Eyed
Parent   Parent

Because the allele for brown eyes is the dominant one, the result here is that any child of these parents will have brown eyes. These offspring, however, would not, as you see, carry the pure strain of the trait. Rather, because they would each receive one dominant brown-eyed allele and one recessive blue-eyed allele, the offspring would be heterozygous (each would possess both forms of the eye-color gene) and could still pass on a recessive allele, in turn, to their children.

And what happens when two heterozygous brown-eyed people, in the course of human events, meet, fall in love, marry, and have children? Science can't predict everything that will happen to this family, but it can still predict eye color. Again, both parents will pass one of their two eye-color genes on to each of their children. But because they each carry two different genes, there are different potential outcomes in the four possible pairings:

Heterozygous Brown-Eyed Parents

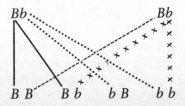

In one of the four pairings, an offspring would carry a pure strain of the dominant brown-eyed trait (*BB*); in two of the pairings the result is a heterozygous brown-eyed child (*Bb*), and in the final possible gene pairing the outcome would be a blue-eyed child (*bb*) who is homozygous for the recessive eye-color trait. That doesn't mean that this couple, if they have four children, will inevitably have one blue-eyed and three brown-eyed kids; rather, it indicates that *any one child* of the couple has a 75 percent chance of having brown eyes and a 25 percent chance of having blue eyes.

This simplified scenario also illustrates why a particular trait may "skip" generations and why it may be expressed in one child but not in his or her siblings. For a truly accurate genetic picture, you need to look at your entire family tree.

Diseases with a genetic component, however, do not usually obey so simple a scheme. The human genome is infinitely more complex, with thousands of genes influencing thousands of traits, and often several genes influencing one trait. Still, the same basic truths apply; for practical purposes, this is the essential mechanism by which a predisposition to genetically associated diseases might be inherited. And twenty years ago, scientists began to find tangible evidence that, in many cases, cancer might be one of these diseases.

Discovering the Genetic Link to Cancer

The genetic connection gained real credence in the mid-1970s, when Dr. Harold E. Varmus and Dr. J. Michael Bishop of the University of California at San Francisco identified the presence of *oncogenes,* genes that cause cancer, in all species of animals, from insects to humans. For their discovery, the two doctors won the Nobel Prize in Medicine in 1989.

Oncogenes cause cancer when they produce their protein products in excess. Sometimes that happens when a cell has too many copies of the gene. In other cases, it happens when genes that are meant to inhibit oncogene activity don't do their job.

This class of genes, called *antioncogenes,* or *tumor-suppressor genes,* was being identified by other researchers around the same time Varmus and Bishop were making their oncogene discoveries.

Normally, tumor-suppressor genes keep cell growth and proliferation, necessary to repair worn-out or injured tissues, under control. But if they are lost or absent in the cell, or if they are mutated, they are unable to perform their job and deter the oncogenes. And when they are altered, healthy cells may begin to grow aberrantly, in the worst case eventually becoming malignant tumors.

The mere presence of oncogenes, and absence or mutation of antioncogenes, does not necessarily result in cancer. The influence of an individual gene is generally not strong enough in itself to cause malignancy. Usually, it takes the presence and interaction of several of these genes to result in cancer. Plus, genes don't function in a vacuum. Environmental conditions both within and outside the body play a vital role and can either contribute to or prevent cancer development.

The result is what one scientist has called the "two-hit" theory: People with cancer receive a kind of combination one-two punch from (1) genetic susceptibility and (2) conditions in their environment and lifestyle. Although we can't duck that first hit of hereditary fate, the more we appreciate the extent and limits of its damage, the more we can anticipate the danger of the second, environmental, blow—and can defend ourselves with some clever, healthy lifestyle moves of our own.

So we know about the genetic connection of cancer in general. But what about colorectal cancer specifically? Are there genes that make a person predisposed particularly to this kind of cancer? And are they inherited?

Colorectal Cancer: The Known Genetic Syndromes

The fact is this: Colorectal cancer does indeed run in some families. About 10 to 15 percent of all people with cancer of the large bowel have one or more close relatives (a parent or sibling) who have had the disease. A full 25 percent have some kind of clear family history of cancer.

Having this kind of family background definitely increases your odds of developing colorectal cancer yourself. According to the most recent estimates, with a family history of cancer, your risk for cancer of the large bowel becomes two to three times greater, and the chances that you will develop it at some time in your life rises to 10 to 15 percent.

In some cases, a specific genetic link between colorectal cancer and a family history of cancer can be determined. There are three identified, specific, albeit relatively rare, inherited syndromes that place members of an affected family at significant risk of developing the disease. The cancer resulting from these genetic traits tends to have several characteristics—unusually high occurrence of cancer among family members, early onset of disease, and uncommon location and number of tumors—that distinguish it from the kind of malignancies that the great majority of colorectal cancer patients develop.

Let's take a brief look at these syndromes.

Familial Polyposis Syndrome

Familial polyposis is an inherited condition—affecting about 1 in 7,000 to 8,000 Americans—that causes multiple polyps, some of which are likely to become malignant, to develop in the colon and rectum. Closely related syndromes, including Gardner's syndrome, which affects about 1 in 15,000, as well as Oldfield's and Turcot's syndromes, are often included under the term familial polyposis, and it's likely that all of these are variations of the same genetic defect.

Men and women are equally prone to inherit familial polyposis. The syndrome has little to do with environmental factors; it is passed on in families as an autosomal (nonsex-linked) dominant trait, which means that the child of one affected parent will generally have a 50 percent chance of inheriting the trait. And more than 90 percent of those with the inherited trait develop the disease. The polyps themselves do not start at birth, rather they usually begin growing in adolescence (generally at a later age for Gardner's syndrome).

The inordinate numbers of tumors and their development at an unusually early age clearly distinguish familial polyposis syndrome from the routine nonhereditary appearance of polyps. By the late teens, a person with familial polyposis may have developed hundreds, or even thousands, of adenomas in the large bowel. These polyps grow more frequently, especially early on, in the rectum and lower colon, where the majority of large bowel cancer develops, although people with Gardner's syndrome will commonly have polyps growing throughout the large bowel and often in the right colon.

Because these polyps start appearing very early, if there is a history of familial polyposis in your family, all family members should start to be screened by their early teens.

Along with polyps, cysts and fatty tumors, called *lipomas,* growing beneath the skin or in the bones, especially the jaw bone, may also be present in those who suffer from familial polyposis. Anyone who has these symptoms, and especially if that person also has a family history of polyposis, should immediately be examined for the syndrome and for the presence of any benign or malignant polyps. And very soon, there should be even more direct evidence to analyze. With the recent discovery of the actual gene believed to cause familial polyposis, for example, genetics experts are now in the process of devising a simple blood test that will positively ascertain the presence of the condition.

What's inherited in familial polyposis is not cancer itself, but rather a trait that causes the proliferation of tumors that, in turn, strongly predisposes you to colorectal cancer. You may have multiple polyps without being affected by familial polyposis.

And some families unaffected by familial polyposis nevertheless still have a greater tendency to develop polyps in the large bowel. But this predisposition doesn't involve the proliferation of hundreds of polyps nor does it usually appear so early in life. Again, the presence of a great number of these growths at an early age is a pretty good indication that you carry the genetic disorder.

About one in a hundred people with malignancies in the large bowel has a background of familial polyposis. Left untreated, the risk of colorectal cancer rises progressively with age: by age forty, more than 80 percent of people with familial polyposis will have at least one cancerous tumor; virtually 100 percent by age fifty. In infrequent cases, cancer may even develop in childhood.

Treatment for Familial Polyposis. Because of the great likelihood of eventually developing colorectal cancer, as a preventive measure most people with familial polyposis are strongly advised by physicians to have their colon removed when the condition is first diagnosed, usually by age twenty. This is radical surgery, yes, but it's not as dire as it sounds. To begin with, if the whole large bowel is removed, the risk for colorectal cancer that they would surely develop otherwise is entirely eliminated, and that is good news indeed. Second, the colon and rectum need not both necessarily be removed. About one in five people with familial polyposis do not develop these growths in the rectum. If it is relatively free of polyps, doctors may let the rectum be retained, connecting it in surgery to the lower section of the small intestine (we'll discuss this kind of procedure in detail in chapter 7), which eradicates the need of a colostomy. This has the great advantage of being not nearly as disruptive as removal of the entire bowel; however, it is a controversial method. That's because it leaves the risk that cancer will still develop in the retained rectum—a risk ranging from 5 to 60 percent and increasing over time. So a person with polyposis who has had this operation must be unfailingly diligent about receiving regular examinations—as often as every six months—for polyp growth and development of malignancies in the rectum.

Lynch Syndrome I—Familial Colorectal Cancer Syndrome

The cancer caused by this syndrome is also sometimes called hereditary site-specific nonpolyposis colorectal cancer, which, although an unwieldy term, pretty much describes it. Lynch syndrome I is an inherited trait, unrelated to polyposis, that causes affected family members specifically to develop cancer of the large bowel. The nature of this genetic disorder, and with it the related Lynch syndrome II, is not as well understood as familial polyposis. It is believed to be inherited, like familial polyposis, as an autosomal dominant trait, so the child of an affected parent has about a 50 percent chance of receiving the affected gene. Among those who have inherited the trait, more than 90 percent have been found ultimately to develop cancer of the large bowel.

The four features that often distinguish cancers related to familial colorectal cancer syndrome are

1. A tendency for colorectal cancer to strike several family members and to strike in more than one generation.
2. A tendency for the cancer to develop at a relatively early age, often before age fifty. (This is probably because the affected gene is inherited, thereby giving the cancer a head start—from birth—in its development.)
3. A tendency to develop multiple malignancies in the bowel.
4. A tendency for malignant tumors to grow in the right colon (remember that the majority of colorectal cancers develop in the rectum, or left side of the colon).

Who Is at Risk? Because the indications aren't precise, it's often difficult to determine with certainty the presence of the familial colorectal cancer syndrome in your family, especially if the medical history of family members is sketchy. Nevertheless, if you have at least one *first-degree relative*—a parent, sibling, or child—with colorectal cancer, current statistics suggest that alone means your immediate family is three to five times more likely than the average family to be carrying familial colorectal cancer syndrome. (More distant blood relations have less of an influence, and spouses and other nonblood relatives, because they don't share your genetic background, do not count here.) Keep in mind, though, that the syndome is a rare one, and it's still highly probable that it doesn't run in your family. But if the cancer experiences of your relatives share several of the characteristics listed above, then it becomes increasingly possible that your family is affected by this genetic disorder. That's why it's so important to know as much about the health background of each relative across the past couple of generations. (We'll explain how to go about this later in this chapter.) It's equally important, especially if you suspect a genetic link, to report this family background to your doctor. That way, he or she, often in consultation with specialists, can make a determination about the syndrome's possible presence and then develop with you the proper screening and prevention program for you and your family.

Lynch Syndrome II—Familial Cancer Syndrome

Also called hereditary adenocarcinomatosis, this is a more general genetic disorder affecting certain families that have a history of several kinds of cancer in addition to cancer of the large bowel. Although most of the noncolorectal cancers associated with *Lynch syndrome II* affect women only, men are just as likely to inherit this trait.

Familial cancer syndrome is also considered an autosomal dominant trait. Like Lynch syndrome I, there are no unique symptoms per se, but the disorder is often characterized by:

1. Multiple family members, across several generations, who
    have developed various forms of cancer.
2. Occurrence, in the family, of cancers of the breast, ovaries,
    and especially the uterus (endometrial cancer), as well as
    cancer of other areas of the gastrointestinal system, in
    addition to cancer of the large bowel.
3. Unusually early onset of cancer.
4. Tendency for colorectal cancer to develop in the right
    colon.

Again, if you know that one or more of these characteristics
is present in your family, even though they do not definitively
indicate the presence of Lynch syndrome II, you and your doctor
should consider the possibility that you have a hereditary link
to cancer. As you can see, familial cancer syndrome shares many
of the same traits as Lynch syndrome I, and the two are thought
to be variations of the same genetic mutation.

With Lynch syndrome II, however, members of your family
are far more likely to develop the other forms of cancer listed
above as well as colorectal cancer. Multiple primary cancers, in
fact, may develop in as many as one-half of the people who are
affected by familial cancer syndrome, while normally less than
3 to 5 percent of patients with one kind of cancer will go on to
develop cancer in another part of the body. And unlike Lynch
syndrome I, this genetic disorder does not even necessarily affect
the large bowel. Oftentimes, family members who carry the trait
will not develop colorectal cancer at all, although it, along with
uterine cancer, is the most common site for a malignancy to
occur.

Sporadic Cancer: A Hereditary Link?

The great majority of people with colorectal cancer—probably
close to 85 percent—have what is called *sporadic cancer,* a

malignancy uninfluenced by any clearly identified disorder. Nevertheless, for many of these individuals, there is also evidence of a hereditary link. A lot of people who develop cancer of the large bowel have a family history of the disease, yet there's no strong indication for the presence of one of the three genetic syndromes listed here. In some families that clearly don't suffer from familial polyposis, for example, there is still a decided tendency to develop polyps in the colon or rectum. And although there may be a high incidence of colorectal cancer among first-degree relatives, it may not be matched by unusually early onset of the disease or a tendency to form in the right colon, or any of the other physical markers for the Lynch syndromes.

Still, the increased probability of developing cancer if a close relative has had the disease—again, a two to three times greater risk—gives a powerful indication that a genetic influence, perhaps contributing a less certain susceptibility, may yet be playing a key role.

A Study of Spouses and Blood Relatives

One way to determine if there is a genetic component is by looking at how close the link is between the presence of cancer or benign tumors in the large bowel and a family history of colorectal cancer in a sufficiently large group of people and by verifying that environmental factors are not the only ones at work in sporadic disease. That's what Dr. Lisa Cannon-Albright, Dr. Randall W. Burt, and their colleagues at the University of Utah did, announcing the landmark results of their study in 1989 (*New England Journal of Medicine*, 321:1290–1292, 1989).

There had been several previous studies showing that close relatives of people who have had colorectal cancer have an increased risk of developing the disease. But none of them had demonstrated that the connection was so specific and pronounced that a clear pattern of genetic inheritance could be seen.

For their study, the University of Utah researchers needed a large, easily accessible group of people whose genealogies (family histories) were well known. They couldn't do much better than with people right there in Utah, a state whose large Mormon population is keenly interested in genealogy. The doctors also needed to compare the individuals in their study with a control population, people who shared, as similarly as possible, the lifestyles and demographics of the subjects, but not their predisposition to colorectal cancer. Thus a possible environmental contribution could be determined. For this control group, the subjects' spouses were used. They weren't, of course, blood relations, but they did share the same environment. If in a particularly large number of these couples, one spouse developed cancer, or benign tumors, while the other didn't, then it could be concluded that there were indeed factors other than the environment that contributed to cancer development. And if, in significant numbers, the spouses who did develop tumors had a family history of colorectal cancer, then the presence of an inheritance factor was likely.

The University of Utah study involved 640 people from thirty-four families. All the individuals in the study were white and of predominantly British and Northern European heritage. The families chosen were not affected by familial polyposis or the familial cancer syndromes. But they either had one member who had developed an adenomatous polyp, benign or malignant, or a cluster of close blood relatives with a personal history of colorectal cancer. Then the subjects were screened for tumors in the large bowel. Did those individuals with polyps have a family history of the cancer? Did those with affected family members have polyps themselves? And did the subjects' spouses have a presence or absence of polyps in similar patterns?

The results: A clear pattern of inheritance emerged, a pattern so strong that the doctors concluded there indeed exists a gene (or genes) that if inherited, makes an individual susceptible to either benign or malignant tumors in the large bowel. At least 53 percent of the study's subjects who developed either benign or malignant tumors in the large bowel were found to have this genetic susceptibility to the disease. And from the data obtained, the researchers used computer modeling to determine that most cases of colorectal cancer may be directly influenced by a genetic hereditary predisposition.

Furthermore, the University of Utah doctors were able to conclude that approximately one in three white Americans, a significantly higher proportion than had been previously estimated, have this genetic susceptibility to cancer of the large bowel. Again, computer modeling was used to calculate that a gene promoting colorectal cancer is likely to be present in 32 percent of people in the same demographic group nationwide.

But an individual's fate in regard to the disease is never preordained. *The study does not suggest in the least that all 32 percent with the genetic susceptibility, or even the majority of them, will eventually get cancer.* Many of the subjects in the study who had a solid family background of colorectal cancer and who seemed likely to have inherited the gene did not develop cancer—or even benign polyps. What it does point out is that perhaps as many as one-third of white Americans are at higher risk of developing colorectal cancer because of the hereditary factor alone. Your genes may set you up for the possibility of developing colorectal cancer, and you may have little control over that. But the variable under your control—the key influence that can determine whether cancer will actually develop—appears once again to be your environment. The University of Utah study reinforced the two-hit theory, that genetic and environmental influences interact to foster the formation of benign polyps in the large bowel—and their transformation into malignant ones.

The study's final conclusion—and one equally important for our purposes—is that anyone with at least one first-degree relative who has had colorectal cancer should consider himself or herself at high risk for the disease as well and, therefore, should probably begin regular screening for the disease even ten years before the general population, by age forty, and in some cases even earlier.

The University of Utah study also identified in a very systematic way the hereditary component of sporadic cancer. But even with its now seemingly clear genetic link, sporadic colorectal cancer is not yet characterized as a genetic disorder. That's because this trait gives affected persons only a *susceptibility*—strongly influenced by outside forces—to the disease. This is the kind of predisposition to cancer we're most likely to carry, and it's the kind where we have abounding influence over our fate.

In other words, you can still make choices in the way you live your life that can significantly reduce your chances of getting cancer. For those who are susceptible, it really pays to educate yourself and your family about the kind of diet and lifestyle practices that can contribute to cancer development—and the kind that can prevent it from ever developing. You can begin with chapter 4 of this book.

Genetics Research: The Frontiers

It's been said that the final, categorical proof of the genetic link in colorectal cancer would be the identification of the actual cancer-causing gene or genes. And with those genes isolated, we may, in the future, be able to prevent certain hereditary forms of the disease altogether. Well, the future, as they say, has already begun to arrive.

Over the past decade and a half, since the presence of oncogenes in humans was first discovered, more than sixty of them have been identified. Several groups of genetic researchers have been concentrating specifically on colorectal cancer, and they have made some momentous advances. One example: Individuals can now be tested for the presence of the gene that causes familial polyposis (ask your doctor about this procedure if you suspect polyposis runs in your family).

In 1988, scientists in Japan led by Dr. Yusuke Nakamura of the Tokyo Cancer Institute presented evidence identifying several chromosomes that hold a group of tumor-suppressor genes whose loss or alteration is believed to cause a hereditary susceptibility to cancer of the large bowel. The findings confirmed the widely held belief that most colorectal cancers require more than one gene mutation. They also suggested that the number of mutated genes may not only determine whether a person will develop cancer but also may determine the course and probable outcome of the cancer—how quickly and widely it will spread.

Other investigators in the past two and a half years have been able to home in on the culpable genes even further. They've done this by carefully analyzing tissues from a large number of cancerous tumors and benign polyps found in the colon and rectum. By examining the chromosomes of the tissue cells, they have been able to isolate specific changes in the genes that seem to transform a healthy cell, or a benign tumor, into a malignant one. They have found that certain chromosomes seemed to be regularly associated with various stages of cancer development. Lost or mutated genes located on chromosome 5, for example, were often detected in tissue cells from benign polyps, whereas gene alterations on chromosomes 17 and 18 were only observed in cancerous tissue.

The big breakthrough came from a team of researchers at Johns Hopkins University led by Dr. Bert Vogelstein and Dr. Eric Fearon. They concluded that the most serious forms of colorectal cancer require mutations of a group of five to seven specific genes, at least one of them an oncogene, that work together to cause the disease to grow and spread. And they have proceeded to identify three of the tumor-suppressor genes in this group that, when damaged, will encourage the development of colorectal cancer.

The first gene they isolated, in June 1989, located on chromosome 17 (*Journal of the American Medical Association,* 261:3099–3103, 1989), has now been solidly identified as a prime culprit in familial cancer syndrome and is suspected to be involved in the development of cancer of the lung and kidney, too. A second gene was discovered in January 1990 (*Science,* 247:49–56, 1990), which may also be associated with the Lynch syndromes, because it is located on the same part of chromosome 18 as the gene linked to these inherited disorders. This finding gives still another strong hint that the genetic mutations involved in sporadic colorectal cancer are often inherited as well. And through a collaboration between the Johns Hopkins group, Dr. Nakamura's team at the Tokyo Cancer Institute, and researchers from the University of Utah headed by Dr. Raymond White, yet another gene believed to affect sporadic cancer of the large bowel was disclosed in May 1991 (*Science,* 251:1386–1390, 1991).

Then, in August 1991, after years of examining chromosome 5, where the defect related to familial polyposis was putatively located, those same teams of scientists finally pinpointed the actual gene believed to cause the trait (*Science,* 253:661–668, 1991 and *Cell,* 66:pp. 589–613, 1991), and it has been the most exciting discovery yet. For while the first three genes isolated chiefly are involved in more advanced stages of malignancy, this one, profoundly damaged in people with familial polyposis, also appears to be the very gene responsible for the initiation of cancer in the large bowel. Mild hereditary defects or environmental mutations of the gene too weak in themselves to cause a condition as extreme as familial polyposis nevertheless can still trigger the transformation of healthy cells on the intestinal lining into polyps. The implications of this finding on the early detection and treatment of colorectal cancer, as we'll see, could be enormous.

But the impact of this discovery depends on whether the defective form of the gene actually does appear in most colonic tumors, and that, although the early signs are encouraging, remains to be seen. Mutations of the first two genes located by the Johns Hopkins team were not always present in the cancerous tissues they studied.

That, too, however, tells us a lot, further indicating that the wide variations in the course of colorectal cancer result from variations in the specific mutations present. The gene on chromosome 18, for example, was found to be missing or damaged in about 70 percent of the malignant tissue samples and was associated in particular with cancer that had metastasized. While they haven't yet established a definitive correlation, the Johns Hopkins investigators have been able to suggest from this information that the absence or mutation of this particular gene will accelerate the cancer to its most dangerous stage.

What Does This Mean for You?

Even though you'd need to possess several of these mutated genes to develop this grave kind of colorectal cancer, inheriting any one of them leaves you particularly vulnerable to the disease. That's because a potentially cancerous cell will already have a head start, needing one fewer gene to be damaged over the whole course of your lifetime.

But the good news is that with the knowledge that has been gained about the particular genetic components of colorectal cancer, scientists have already begun to be able to combat the disease more effectively than ever before. Genetics experts are starting to predict the course of disease—its likelihood of developing as well as the speed and extent of its growth—based on the particular combination of damaged genes that an individual carries. Perhaps soon we will be able to perform a genetic test for susceptibility before any signs or symptoms of the disease appear, just as fetuses are tested for Tay-Sachs disease and Down's syndrome.

The discovery of that one crucial tumor-suppressor gene on chromosome 5 could likely result in remarkable advances and changes in early detection of malignancies. After more careful study to confirm that the mutation is indeed present in the majority of colonic tumors, scientists may ultimately be able to develop an inexpensive and highly accurate diagnostic test that would catch colorectal cancer from the beginning—simply by determining whether the telltale mutation was present in intestinal cells that appear in a stool or blood sample. And investigators will undoubtedly soon begin to explore the potential of gene splicing in colorectal cancer treatment, as they have with other kinds of cancers, inserting undamaged tumor-suppressor genes into cancerous cells to attempt to block or slow their growth.

All of the current genetics research offers enormous possibilities, but also carries enormous implications. "The day may be near when individuals can request a personalized genetic map with all of their health 'land mines' demarcated," says Dr. Nancy Wexler, president of the Hereditary Disease Foundation. The Human Genome Project may hasten that day. This fifteen-year, $3 billion enterprise, sponsored by the National Institutes of Health and the Department of Energy, is attempting to determine the identity and location of each of our 100,000 genes. The success of this ambitious project could enable this kind of genetic profile to become commonplace.

Doctors of the not-too-distant future may be able to analyze our individual "genetic maps" to determine not only our likelihood of developing certain diseases like colorectal cancer but also the particular environmental factors that are most likely to encourage or discourage its development. You can guess the value and magnitude of this information: It will allow us to practice the best and most effective kind of preventive medicine.

Does this impending new knowledge have any drawbacks? Perhaps. It will provide far more information about the health problems we will face in the future—and pass on to the next generation—than any of us are used to. Do you always want to know what's in store for you? How and when you're likely to die? Would you want to know if you will be confronting some kind of incurable, debilitating illness long before you're old? And would you want your prospective employer—or insurance company—to know? How would your decision to have children be affected? Or your relationship with the children you already have?

Maybe that all is a bit excessively dire. First of all, few genetic disorders bring the tragic inevitability of conditions like Tay-Sachs or Huntington's disease. Because most genetic conditions involve several genes, in addition to the influence of environmental factors, it's highly unlikely you'll be able to get a simple yes or no prediction, let alone a specific pronouncement, about how your life span will be affected. But you will be able to have a clearer picture of the genetically related diseases to which you may be vulnerable—and of the ways you'll be able to fight them.

In the case of colorectal cancer, a little more knowledge is always a good thing. For, armed with that knowledge, you are in the best position to wage a three-pronged attack on the disease:

- Diet and other lifestyle changes to decrease or eliminate the chances of the disease developing.
- Regular screening to detect dysplasia or polyps before they become cancerous or to catch a tumor when it has just begun to turn malignant.
- Early treatment of the disease if it does develop, offering the great likelihood that you will go on to live a full, normal, and long life.

How to Begin Your Own Search: Tracing Your Family History

While genetic research is advancing, there is much you can do in the meantime to learn about your possible hereditary susceptibility to colorectal cancer. Look for some answers on your own.

One way to do it is by constructing a family genogram. That's simply a fancy term for a family tree that notes information about inheritable traits, conditions, and syndromes of relatives across several generations. You've probably already done an informal variation of a family tree, perhaps as part of a school social studies project or to explain arcane lineage details to your children or someone marrying into the fold ("Uncle Henry isn't actually an uncle, he's more of a second cousin once removed—or is it first cousin twice removed?") or because you were inspired by watching *Roots*. A genogram requires a little more detail of a somewhat more somber and occasionally obscure nature: the diseases and ailments from which family members present and past have suffered and died.

For our purposes, we're interested in the incidence of cancer of the large bowel, of course, but also of some related conditions as well. But we begin with the basics, and the construction of a family tree. For the diagram, you can use the standard genogram symbols recommended by the Task Force of the North American Primary Care Research Group and described in *Genograms in Family Assessment* by Monica McGoldrick and Randy Gerson (W. W. Norton & Co., 1985).

Start with you and your siblings. You may want to draw a double line around yourself so you can easily spot where you fit in to the increasingly complicated picture as the diagram gets fuller and busier.

Then go on to your parents, also filling in their siblings—your

= Male (living)   = Female (living)

= Male (deceased)   = Female (deceased)

= Marriage   = Children

= Twins (boys)   = Adopted Children

aunts and uncles. For a more complete picture, you may want to include their children—your cousins—and then continue going back as far as you can, to your parents' parents, their siblings, their parents, and so on, until you have an intricate, bushy, network of branches and layers. Fill in everyone's name and year of birth as well as the year of death for everyone who has died. (If you wish to identify your children's possible risk of developing colorectal cancer, you might want to do a separate genogram for them, which will include their other parent's side of the family as well as your own.)

Now add the information that is relevant to your search for a possible hereditary link to colorectal cancer. As we've seen, it's not only valuable to know whether a family member has had the disease, but also to know many of the specifics of the disease in order to determine a potential genetic connection. Obviously, the details will be easier to obtain from relatives who are still alive. The picture will undoubtedly get murkier the further back you go, but that's not really such a problem. It's the information about your first-degree relatives (siblings, parents, children) that is most relevant to your inherited risk of the disease. Nevertheless, any information about previous generations or other branches of the family is helpful in filling out the whole genetic picture.

Your Genogram Checklist

Throughout this chapter, we've discussed the ways colorectal cancer runs in some families, the traits that tend to characterize cancer that may have resulted from an inherited predisposition. The presence or absence of these conditions among your relatives is what you want to find out and note here. To summarize, as you collect the information for your family genogram, here's what to ask about and record:

- Any incidence of cancer of the colon or rectum.
- Where in the large bowel the cancer developed (if known).

- Whether cancer developed at multiple sites (if known).
- The age at which the cancer was diagnosed (remember that under fifty suggests greater likelihood of a genetic connection).
- Any recurrence of colorectal cancer.
- Any incidence of cancers of other parts of the gastrointestinal tract or of the ovaries, uterus, or breast.
- The age at which *those* cancers were diagnosed.
- Any incidence of polyps in the colon or rectum.
- The age at which the polyps were discovered.
- The location of the polyps and whether multiple polyps were found (if known).
- Any incidence of familial polyposis syndrome (Gardner's, Oldfield's, or Turcot's syndromes).
- Any incidence of inflammatory bowel disease (particularly ulcerative colitis, but also Crohn's disease) and when the condition was diagnosed.

List this information, as completely as possible, next to each affected relative. And fill in the facts as you learn them—don't wait until every question is answered, every detail uncovered. You may never know all the particulars for every member of your family, but simply by gathering together the facts readily known in this kind of diagram, you may be able to see a pattern emerge.

As you proceed to collect this information and add it to your genogram, it will begin to look something like Figure 2.

Interpreting the Results

The information you gather in your family genogram is often confusing, even frequently peppered with contradictions. In examining Elizabeth's genogram (Figure 2), there does seem to be a pattern on her father's side of the family, even a possible indication of familial cancer syndrome, although she shouldn't

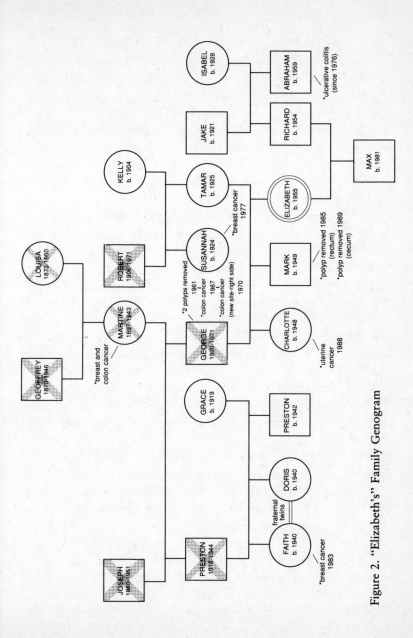

Figure 2. "Elizabeth's" Family Genogram

jump to conclusions and make the diagnosis herself. Her father developed colon cancer at age forty-seven, a relatively young age for the disease—although not *so* unusually early in life that the presence of the syndrome can definitely be pinpointed—and a second malignancy developed three years later, on the right side of the colon where cancer resulting from the syndrome is more likely to occur. Elizabeth's paternal grandmother had colon cancer too, and breast cancer as well. Her father's brother showed no sign of a disease, although that may be because he died at age twenty-six in World War II, before a malignancy caused by genetic predisposition developed or was seen. One of this uncle's daughters was diagnosed with breast cancer at age forty-three; however, because this disease is hardly unusual (it's by far the most common form of cancer among women the age of Elizabeth's cousin), that can't necessarily be attributed to the syndrome. Among Elizabeth's own siblings, the signs are more ominous. Her sister developed uterine cancer, a disease particularly associated with the syndrome, by age forty; and before age forty, her brother has already had two polyps, including one growing on the right colon. While these occurrences might simply be a coincidence, Elizabeth should, nevertheless, certainly be watchful, and although she herself is not yet forty, she should probably begin a regular screening program, as we'll discuss in chapter 6.

Your own genogram may yield much more vague results. The point is, you don't make a genogram expecting to unravel all the mysteries of your hereditary background. It's meant, rather, to give you a general overview. And that alone is invaluable. Merely by knowing you have one or more first-degree relatives who has had colorectal cancer gives you a great deal of information. You will then know, as we've seen, that you should consider yourself—and possibly your children, if you have them—at high risk of the disease. The more you become aware from the genogram that colorectal cancer, and related conditions, run in the family, the more you become aware how important it is to be on your guard.

If there's no pattern at all—if the entire tree appears blissfully free of any connection to colorectal cancer, then so much the better, although don't let that lure you into a false sense of invincibility. Cancer of the large bowel does not *require* an inherited predisposition, and given the lifestyle many Americans lead, you could inherit the most pristine genes in the world and still proceed to turn them into insidious things that will destroy your health.

Similarly, even if a very clear pattern does emerge, don't panic. Instead, bring all this information to your doctor, who will help you interpret the findings and design an appropriate screening and prevention program. And you may also want to begin looking closely at the kind of everyday practices you can initiate to reduce your risk.

Questions and Answers

Q: I am adopted, and don't know anything about the background of my biological family. How can I determine my genetic connection to colorectal cancer?

A: The agency that handled your adoption may have maintained records of your biological parents' medical history. So you can try to contact them. But you can't count on the agency having this information, and without it, short of tracking down your biological parents and asking them directly, you may never be able to find out about your family's medical history. But, as we've seen, with the advances in genetic research, the time is perhaps not far off when you will be able to learn from a simple test all kinds of details about your individual genetic makeup, including your susceptibility to colorectal cancer. In the meantime, you should certainly not consider yourself free of any hereditary risk of the disease and might even want to act as though you were at high risk. In both cases, that means following sensible health and lifestyle practices and being screened regularly starting at age forty, or earlier if you develop any symptoms that may indicate the presence of a polyp or malignancy.

Q: Several doctors have reviewed my family's health background, and they say we carry familial cancer syndrome. What should I do?

A: The first thing is not to submit to fear and fatalism. To begin with, although the syndrome may run in your family, there's still a good possibility that you yourself did not inherit it. You will only carry the gene if one of your parents had it, and even then you only stand a 50 percent chance of inheriting it. While that definitely places you at high risk, it's by no means a sure thing. In addition, although a high percentage do, not everyone who carries the gene winds up developing cancer, which suggests that there are environmental influences that may still be necessary for the disorder to be expressed. So you shouldn't assume you have no control over the situation but should be extra conscientious about making the kind of changes in your diet and lifestyle that can help in cancer prevention. It's just as important that your whole family follow a sensitive diet and health program, because your children too, after all, are at risk of carrying the disorder. Also, make sure you are fully aware of the symptoms not only of colorectal cancer but also of the other kinds of cancer—breast, ovarian, cervical, endometrial, and other gastrointestinal cancers—associated with familial cancer, so you know the signs to look for to aid in early detection of those diseases. Finally, be sure to discuss with your doctor a complete game plan involving regular screening for all these cancers, so any malignancies that develop can be caught at their earliest stage. Even with a genetic disorder like familial cancer syndrome, a comprehensive early screening and detection program may well keep you and your family from ever developing cancer.

Q: As far as I know, no one in my family has ever developed colorectal cancer. Should I still be concerned about getting it?

A: Your family background makes it more unlikely that you will develop colorectal cancer, but no one is entirely risk free. In the first place, it's possible you're simply unaware of some episode of cancer of the large bowel in your family. Remember that cancer was long a taboo subject, and people are still reluctant to discuss diseases of the colon and rectum. The death or hospital stay of some relative, particularly from a generation or two past, could have, in "polite company," been attributed to something else, when in reality colorectal cancer was the cause.

Also keep in mind the latest genetic research concerning genes that in combination may make you susceptible to the disease. One of those genes in and of itself may not be sufficient to cause cancer, so families that carry it may never even have a single member affected. But it's possible to inherit a damaged gene from each of your unaffected parents, which will thus put you at far greater risk yourself.

One other thing to remember. No one ever said that a hereditary predisposition is necessary for developing colorectal cancer. Genes can go haywire in a cell just as easily when they're damaged by some outside force as when they're inherited that way. This, once again, is the much trumpeted environmental factor, which we will discuss in the next chapter. Read on to find out about the dietary habits and lifestyle features that can contribute to the development of colorectal cancer, making even someone with a clean hereditary slate potentially vulnerable to the disease—and putting an already high-risk individual at even greater risk.

4

Environmental Factors: Reducing the Risk

Answer these questions to find out what you may be doing—
and what more you could do—to reduce your risk of developing
cancer of the large bowel.

		Score
1.	Do you (successfully) try to limit the amount of fat in your diet?	_____
2.	Are you no more than 10 percent heavier than your ideal weight?	_____
3.	Is your cholesterol level low or moderate?	_____
4.	Do you eat high-fiber foods regularly?	_____
5.	Do you eat plenty of fruits and vegetables?	_____
6.	Do you take care to eat foods high in calcium?	_____
7.	Do you live in a relatively sunny area?	_____

8.   Do you engage in frequent outdoor activities?   _____
9.   Do you exercise regularly?   _____

Now read on to learn exactly how these dietary and lifestyle practices might help influence colorectal cancer prevention.

The First Line of Defense

It can be due to your health background or due to your family background: You and your loved ones may be at increased risk of developing colorectal cancer. That, however, is only the beginning of the story. In the years, sometimes decades, it takes for cancer to develop in the large bowel, there are other factors very much under your control that help—or hinder—malignant activity. All the indications suggest it usually takes a combination of hereditary predisposition and environmental influences to cause colorectal cancer. You can do something about the environmental factors.

Reducing your risk of developing colorectal cancer by making changes in the way you live is your first line of defense against the disease. It begins with your diet.

Because colorectal cancer is, after all, a disease formed in the intestinal tract, it makes sense that the foods we eat might affect cancerous activity. Although the precise relationships are difficult to determine, epidemiologists (doctors who study patterns of diseases) have long associated certain diets with higher incidence of colorectal cancer—a high-fat, low-fiber so-called Western diet in particular. Colorectal cancer, as we've already seen, is far more prevalent in Europe, Australia, and the United States, countries where the Western diet is common. The disease is much rarer in Japan and the Third World, countries where the typical diet contains far less fat and more fiber.

It's clear there is a preponderance of colorectal cancer in certain parts of the world. But couldn't that merely be due to the genetic factor? Statistics suggest otherwise. First-generation Japanese emigrants in Hawaii, for example, who have similar genetic backgrounds to their counterparts still living in Japan but who tend to eat the Western diet, have rates of colorectal cancer similar to the Caucasian population. Vegetarians in the United States have lower rates of the disease than meat-eating Americans. And, as we'll see, numerous studies strongly point to particular substances and nutrients that appear to make a big difference in the progress of colorectal cancer.

There are environmental factors other than diet that seem to make a difference as well. Why do people living in the Northeast, or living in large cities, develop colorectal cancer more often than those in the South or Southwest? What role does exercise play? Do smoking or drinking make a difference?

The potential of simply eating the right combinations of foods to help protect against cancer is startling and extremely exciting. It's also an area, however, particularly susceptible to faddism. But little of what will be discussed here falls into that category. The recommendations in this chapter do not require you to eat unreasonable amounts of any one kind of food or to take massive doses of some miracle substance. Actually, they don't even require you to eat much differently from what any nutritionist would recommend for a well-balanced diet. It just so happens that a healthy low-fat, high-fiber diet appears to have the added benefit of helping to prevent colorectal cancer. While we may not be certain precisely how eating the right kinds of foods—and avoiding others—can discourage cancer development, the evidence increasingly suggests that doing that, in fact, works.

We're continuing to learn more, but we already know a lot. Certainly enough for you to start determining if you and your family are engaging in practices that seem likely to increase your risk of developing colorectal cancer—and certainly enough for you to start making the remarkably simple changes in your lifestyle to protect yourself and your family. Here are the factors that may make the difference.

Fat in the Diet

The rates of colorectal cancer tend to be highest in countries where the typical daily diet is high in fat. In the United States, for example, an average of 40 percent of our total caloric intake is from fat. Compare that with Japan, where colorectal cancer rates are notably low and where fats on average account for only about 10 to 20 percent of the calories the Japanese consume. Consider at the same time that Americans of Japanese descent tend to have a diet about as high in fat as the national average—and wind up developing cancers of the large bowel at pretty much the same rate as other Americans.

Furthermore, studies that monitor groups of people with similar health and family backgrounds have shown time and time again that those whose diets are highest in fat are much more likely—the results have ranged from two to as high as eight times more likely—to develop colorectal cancer. All this has led to a wide acceptance among medical experts that fat is likely to be one of the chief promoting agents of cancer of the large bowel.

Some particularly convincing evidence linking a high-fat diet to colorectal cancer came in December 1990, in a startling report by Dr. Walter Willett of Boston's Brigham and Women's Hospital and his colleagues (*New England Journal of Medicine,* 323:1664–1672, 1990). The team examined the diets of almost 89,000 female nurses between the ages of thirty-four and fifty-nine over a six-year period, by far the largest study of its kind yet conducted. This was part of an even larger national research project by Willett's team, the well-known Nurses' Health Study, that has followed 122,000 subjects since 1976 to learn about connections between diet and disease among American women.

Willett and his coworkers found that the subjects who ate red meat as a main course at least once a day were two and a half times more likely to develop colorectal cancer than those who ate beef, pork, or lamb sparingly or not at all (chicken and fish consumption—meat products significantly lower in fat—was unrelated to any higher rate of malignancy). That finding itself doesn't rule out the possibility that it's the red meat itself, not the fat in it, that contains cancer-causing agents. But when actual animal fat intake was specifically analyzed, those women with the highest levels of animal fat in their diet were found to be nearly twice as likely to develop cancer of the large bowel.

It's not known exactly how digestion of fats can lead to colorectal cancer. In recent years, many popular and widely accepted theories have focused on the connection between the presence of fats in the large intestine and the production of bile acids. Dietary fats may stimulate increased amounts of bile acids (which are necessary to break down and digest the material) in the large bowel. Animal research has confirmed that elevated fat consumption does promote more production of bile in the intestine and found that the introduction of bile acid–binding resins significantly increased the development of large bowel tumors. Also, people with high-fat diets have been found to excrete greater amounts of bile acids in the stool than people whose diets are lower in fat. What's more, people with colorectal cancer have higher levels of bile acids in the feces as well.

In the bowel, these bile acids remove layers of cells from the intestinal lining, cells that need to be replaced. With the increased production of bile caused by steady heavy intake of dietary fats, that cell turnover may be particularly rapid. And those newly formed and quickly growing cells can be especially vulnerable to cancer-causing agents. Dietary fats may also cause the production of carcinogens themselves when they interact with bile salts, as well as bacteria living in the lumen, or bowel channel. These threatening substances then can proceed to attack the cells developing on the intestinal walls. And don't forget a more obvious connection between dietary fat and carcinogenic substances: The animal fat we consume frequently contains many fat soluble chemicals, like dioxin and PCBs, that may be cancer causing too.

The good news is that it probably takes years of exposure to carcinogenic agents for colorectal cancer to develop. So there's a lot you can start doing now to reduce that exposure: reduce the contact in your body between modified fats and bowel tissue—and thus reduce your risk of getting the disease. That means reducing the fat in your diet.

Americans seem to be more conscious now than ever of the importance of a low-fat diet as an integral part of good general health. Yet, on a national level, we're not doing such a great job in lowering our fat intake. Actually, it's not very hard to do. Again, on average, some 40 percent of the calories we consume come from fat. The figure should be more like 20 to 30 percent—that is, not only if we want to be healthier in general but if we want to enjoy the low colorectal cancer rates of countries like Japan.

If you are convinced by the other information in this chapter to start eating greater quantities of the food that may protect you against cancer of the large bowel, you're already well on your way. By substituting these healthier food items during meals and snacks for the fattier foods you were previously eating, you will be reducing your fat intake significantly right there.

The heavy presence of animal protein in the typical American diet—usually far exceeding recommended daily requirements—contributes greatly to the fat content. Some of the highest rates of colorectal cancer in the world, in fact, are seen in countries like Australia and New Zealand, as well as the United States, known for their heavy beef consumption. Conversely, Seventh-Day Adventists and other vegetarians have notably low incidences of cancer of the large bowel.

The foods on which you should cut back to reduce your risk of colorectal cancer are all the usual high-fat culprits, foods whose majority of calories come from fats. Let's briefly review them.

HIGH-RISK, HIGH-FAT FOODS

Butter and cheese	Gravy	Mayonnaise
Creamy or oily sauces and salad dressings	Ice cream	Nuts
	Junk food (potato chips, candy, and french fries)	Red meat (especially pork)
Fried foods		

In addition, remember these basic elements of low-fat food preparation:

- Avoid cooking with oil and butter. If you do use oil, olive oil, some research has begun to suggest, may be the best choice. People in Greece and Italy, where olive oil is used extensively, have lower rates of colorectal cancer than other Western European nations, even though the overall average dietary fat intake there is pretty much the same. Bake, broil, or steam instead of frying.
- When you do have meat, choose lean cuts and trim excess fat.
- Remove the fatty skin from chicken.
- Substitute skim or low-fat milk for whole milk.

The Cholesterol Paradox

Reports have shown that people with colorectal cancer actually tend to have low levels of cholesterol in their blood. That doesn't mean, however, as was once feared by some, that low cholesterol commonly causes cancer. (Wouldn't that give us a merry choice—eat plenty of food high in cholesterol and risk heart disease, or avoid those foods . . . and risk cancer.) Rather, it's usually the other way around. Cancer of the large bowel seems to *cause* low cholesterol, possibly because the malignancies use the substance to develop and grow. Some researchers do speculate, nonetheless, that having an exceptionally low cholesterol level may weaken cell membranes, making the cell more vulnerable to carcinogens.

But very few of us have to worry about our cholesterol levels being that low. It's the other extreme that is the far more common problem, and it looks like it's a problem affecting our risk of colorectal cancer as well. It seems—and several studies have demonstrated this—that people with high cholesterol levels have a *greater* chance of someday developing cancer of the large bowel. This may simply be because a high cholesterol level is often indicative of a high-fat diet; the particular connection between cholesterol itself and the promotion of colon and rectal cancer isn't at all certain. But many cancer and nutrition specialists do suspect there is a link.

So you may want to consider that controlling your cholesterol is sensible advice, not only for protecton against heart disease, but also possibly to reduce your risk for colorectal cancer. That means, of course, limiting your intake of foods high in cholesterol, including

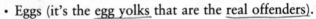

- Eggs (it's the egg yolks that are the real offenders).
- Again, red meat (especially liver and veal).
- Shellfish.
- Foods cooked with oil.
- Butter and cheese.

Obesity

If you're ready to skip this section, thinking to yourself, "Well, sure, maybe I could stand to drop a few pounds, but I wouldn't consider myself *obese,* exactly," read on. Being as little as 10 percent over your recommended weight may signal an increased risk of colorectal cancer, and a great many of us are in that group.

Check yourself against the height and weight tables (Tables

2 and 3) prepared by the Metropolitan Life Insurance Company.

The twelve-year Cancer Prevention Study I, conducted by the American Cancer Society, found that a significantly higher incidence of many kinds of cancer, including cancer of the large bowel, is associated with obesity. And the more overweight you are, the greater likelihood you seem to have of developing cancer. Among people who were 40 percent or more over the average weight for individuals of their height and body frame, the risk of cancer was 55 percent greater for women and 35 percent greater for men than people of normal weight. These subjects had higher death rates from colorectal cancer as well.

It's unclear whether the heightened colorectal cancer risk linked with obesity comes from the amount and kind of food eaten, or from the extra weight and body fat. It may be that eating large amounts of food makes it likelier that cells in the bowel will be exposed to carcinogens more often. Or it may be because what has made you overweight is a poor diet heavy in fats and sugars and low in fiber, vitamins, and other nutrients. It's also possible your high caloric intake has given you a faster metabolic rate, which may increase rampant cell division and multiplication, and subsequently raise the chances of cell mutation. Furthermore, like the animal fat you consume, your own body fat can store cancer-causing substances—to which you're exposed in your food, air, and water—that may initiate malignant activity.

Obesity is more definitely implicated in cancers of the breast, female reproductive organs, and prostate than in cancer of the large bowel. But it's still quite conceivable that weight reduction itself will help protect you against the disease. Certainly engaging in the kinds of practical endeavors, like regular exercise and a low-fat, sensible nutritional program (we're not talking about fad diets—consult your doctor), that will cause you to lose excess weight is a sound course to reduce your chances of developing colorectal cancer.

Table 2. Desired Weights of Men Aged Twenty-five and Over

Height	Small Frame	Medium Frame	Large Frame
5'2"	128–134	131–141	138–150
5'3"	130–136	133–143	140–153
5'4"	132–138	135–145	142–156
5'5"	134–140	137–148	144–160
5'6"	136–142	139–151	146–164
5'7"	138–145	142–154	149–168
5'8"	140–148	145–157	152–172
5'9"	142–151	148–160	155–176
5'10"	144–154	151–163	158–180
5'11"	146–157	154–166	161–184
6'0"	149–160	157–170	164–188
6'1"	152–164	160–174	168–192
6'2"	155–168	164–178	172–197
6'3"	158–172	167–182	176–202
6'4"	162–176	171–187	181–207

Table 3. Desired Weights of Women Aged Twenty-five and Over

Height	Small Frame	Medium Frame	Large Frame
4'10"	102–111	109–121	118–131
4'11"	103–113	111–123	120–134
5'0"	104–115	113–126	122–137
5'1"	106–118	115–129	125–140
5'2"	108–121	118–132	128–143
5'3"	111–124	121–135	131–147
5'4"	114–127	124–138	134–151
5'5"	117–130	127–141	137–155
5'6"	120–133	130–144	140–159
5'7"	123–136	133–147	143–163
5'8"	126–139	136–150	146–167
5'9"	129–142	139–153	149–170
5'10"	132–145	142–156	152–173
5'11"	135–148	145–159	155–176
6'0"	138–151	148–162	158–179

Fiber

Since the early 1970s, we've been hearing how adding fiber to our diets can offer a variety of almost astounding health benefits. And exhaustive animal research, human studies, and anecdotal information over the last two decades have continued to indicate that, at least when it comes to colorectal cancer prevention, fiber really does live up to its hype.

Fiber is actually a generic term covering several categories of material contained in the cells of plants. Often we use the terms fiber and roughage interchangeably, but roughage is only one type of fiber. Technically, fiber itself is the chemical substance that makes up plant cell walls, but other substances found in plant starches, like gums, are generally considered fiber as well. Crude fiber is this material in its original form. Dietary fiber generally refers to the remnants of this material contained in the food we eat that can't be broken down by enzymes during digestion.

Left undigested and sent along with the remains of the other food we've consumed into the large intestine, dietary fiber helps in the formation and passage of waste material. In the colon, it absorbs many times its weight in water, both softening and increasing the bulk of the forming stool. That sends fecal material moving more swiftly through the bowel, preventing constipation. At the same time, fiber also helps to pass other lingering and possibly harmful substances like bile acids out of the intestine.

Fiber has long been known to be an essential part of a good diet. But only fairly recently has the connection between fiber and decreased colorectal cancer risk been suspected. In 1974, British physicians Neil Painter and Denis Burkitt published a report noting that people living in regions of the world where the incidence of colorectal cancer was low tended to eat fiber-rich diets. Painter and Burkitt studied the dietary patterns of several African groups and found an extremely high consumption of fiber among many of them, regularly as high as 50 to

250 grams per day. That's far more than the 8 to 12 grams the typical American eats daily. Painter and Burkitt also pointed out the exceptionally low rates for cancer of the large bowel in these countries. In Nigeria, for example, only about 1 in 700 people ever develop the disease, as opposed to the much higher 1 in 20 chance we have here in the United States.

Right there the evidence seemed pretty convincing. But many researchers noted that high-fiber diets also tended to be low-fat diets; that's certainly the case in Africa. So couldn't it be merely the lack of fat, already believed to have a key effect on the development of large bowel cancer, that led to the lower incidence of the disease in those countries?

Further studies showed that the connection between high-fiber diets and lower rates of colorectal cancer could be seen even in areas where the diet was high in fat as well. Finland is an excellent example. The typical Finnish diet is rather high in fat, about the same amount as in the other Scandinavian countries. But it also, especially in rural areas of Finland where unrefined grain products are a staple, contains much more fiber. For example, the average Finn has been found to eat about 31 grams of fiber per day; the average Dane, 17 grams. And what about the 1984–1986 death rates for colorectal cancer? In Finland it was 17.5 per 100,000; in Denmark, 38.5. Finland's incidence rate for the disease is also only about one-third the rate of the United States, where our diet is lower in fat—but also much lower in fiber.

In countries with a high incidence of colorectal cancer, it appeared that fiber might make a lot of difference. Paul Rozen and his fellow doctors at the Tel Aviv Medical Center, Israel, studied the diets of hundreds of Israelis both with and without colorectal cancer. They found that the subjects who had, or would later develop, cancer of the large bowel tended to eat fiber-rich foods far less often than their cancer-free counterparts.

But the most conclusive evidence thus far came in a study released in 1989 (*Journal of the National Cancer Institute,*

81:1290–1297, 1989). It is the first solid evidence, in fact, that adding fiber to the diet has a direct, beneficial affect on people at high risk of colorectal cancer. Led by Dr. Jerome DeCosse and Dr. Helen Miller of the Memorial Sloane Kettering Cancer Center, and Dr. Martin Lesser of the North Shore University Hospital in New York, the investigation involved fifty-eight people with familial polyposis. As a result of the disease, these subjects had already had their colon removed, but they still retained the rectum, where multiple polyps continued to develop and grow.

The fifty-eight people were asked to go on a regimen where, every day for four years, they would each eat two servings of cereal from an unmarked box. Half were given a cereal extremely rich in fiber—11.5 grams per serving (the cereal used was Kellogg's All-Bran, but any cereal with the equivalent fiber content would likely have the same effect), which alone is double the average amount of fiber Americans consume daily. The other half was given a look-alike low-fiber cereal.

All the subjects were examined every three months. Each rectal polyp found was counted and measured. The results: Those given the high-fiber cereal who adhered most closely to the regimen had a decided tendency to develop fewer polyps. What's more, the polyps that had previously developed were far more likely to have shrunk in size. And that means a reduced risk of cancer. Those given the low-fiber cereal, on the other hand, showed no such tendencies. (As a sidelight, but a significant further implication of fat as a promoter of malignant activity, subjects who ate a high-fat diet were more likely to have greater numbers— and faster growth—of polyps.)

A milestone in nutritional and cancer research, this study focused on familial polyposis patients, but for anyone at high risk of colorectal cancer, the results are particularly significant—and encouraging. We now have strong evidence that adding fiber to the diet can directly inhibit precancerous activity.

How might dietary fiber work to hinder the progress of cancer? One theory, first advanced by Painter and Burkitt in

their 1974 study, suggested that the presence of fiber—by helping to speed material, including fats, through the intestine—
reduces the time that carcinogens would have to form and thus
limits the contact these substances have with cells along the
bowel wall. That, then, limits their ability as well to cause those
cells to mutate. It's also believed that dietary fiber, by increasing
stool bulk, may also act to dilute carcinogens, reducing their
concentration—and thus potency—in the stool. And fiber may
even alter the nature and behavior of bacteria in the bowel,
diminishing their potential for forming other possible cancer-
causing agents. Plus, remember that fiber also helps to dilute
and eliminate bile acids from the intestine, and these acids may
initiate and promote malignant activity. This is one other way,
in fact, that fiber may actually directly counteract the harmful
effect of dietary fat.

   That doesn't mean you can just eat all the fat you like as long
as you get enough fiber. The best course, to be sure, is to both
reduce your fat intake *and* increase the amount of fiber you get
in your diet. But, although it's not difficult to do, you do have
to take care that you are indeed getting the proper amount. Most
Americans, after all, don't. The daily fiber intake among Americans, again, averages only from 8 to 12 grams. It should be
much higher: the National Cancer Institute recommends we
should get from 20 to 30 (but no more than 35) grams of fiber
per day. And what a difference the extra fiber can make! The
Department of Health and Human Services estimates that a high-
fiber, low-fat diet could reduce the number of colorectal cancer
cases by 30 percent. And the National Cancer Institute calculates
that if all Americans ate the recommended 20 to 30 grams of
fiber daily, colorectal cancer rates in this country could fall by
up to 50 percent.

   But fiber, as we've said, is a very broad term. And different
kinds of fiber act in our bodies in different ways. So what kinds
are the most helpful in cancer prevention? The research up to
this point suggests that insoluble fibers, like cellulose and bran
fiber, may be more effective at inhibiting cancer-causing activity,

and even, as the 1989 polyposis study showed, at reducing the size and development of polyps, than other kinds of fiber. Foods rich in these substances include fruits (such as apples, pears, and rhubarb), vegetables (like carrots, lima beans, peas, and brussels sprouts), and nuts (although these can be high in fat, so eat them in moderation) as well as, of course, whole grain breads and all- or high-bran cereals like the kind used in the 1989 study (Table 4).

But nutritionists and other medical professionals regularly recommend you eat foods rich in *all* types of fiber. That encompasses a wide variety of items beyond just bran. It includes, in addition to the foods already mentioned, fruits like berries, dates, bananas, plums, avocados, papayas, nectarines, and tangerines as well as dried apricots, figs, prunes, and raisins. And it also includes vegetables like squash, broccoli, pumpkin, unpeeled potatoes, and especially beans (although they are part of a balanced diet, lettuce and other leafy vegetables actually contain far less fiber than you might imagine). Don't forget legumes, seeds, brown rice, and grains (like oats, buckwheat, bulgur, and stone-ground wheat), which—because they are in coarser form—may be more beneficial than whole wheat flour.

Take a look at Table 4 for a more complete list of the fiber content of various foods. You can see you have many options indeed beyond an all-bran cereal for making your diet fiber rich, and you should not, in any event, try to get all your daily fiber from one source. Again, it is recommended that you obtain your daily fiber from a variety of sources (preferably those foods low in fat and rich in other nutrients as well). In general, two to three servings of fruits and vegetables a day, together with some whole grain (rather than refined) breads and cereals, should give you the fiber you need. (In preparing fruits and vegetables, remember that many are best eaten raw or lightly cooked, with skins, for maximum nutritional value. Avoid boiling or overcooking, as many important vitamins and nutrients can be lost in the cooking process.)

Table 4. Fiber Content of Foods.

Fiber Content of Fruit

Fruit	dietary fiber (gms)
blackberries (½ cup)	5
prunes (4)	4
apple w/ skin (1 avg)	4
raisins (¼ cup)	3
rhubarb (½ cup cooked)	3
strawberries (1 cup)	3
raspberries (½ cup)	3
pear w/ skin (1 avg)	3
orange (1 med)	3
blueberries (½ cup)	2
dates (3)	2
apricots (3 med. fresh)	2
banana (2 avg)	2
peach w/ skin (1 avg)	2

Fiber Content of Crackers

Cracker	dietary fiber (gms)
Ry-Krisp Ralston (2 triple crackers)	2
Fiber Rich Bran (1)	3
Wasa Fiber Plus (1)	3
Finn crisp (2)	2
Fiber crisp bread (2)	2

Fiber Content of Cereals

Cereal (1 oz. serving)	dietary fiber (gms)
All-Bran w/ extra fiber (Kellogg)	13
Fiber One (General Mills)	12
All-Bran (Kellogg)	9
100% Bran (Nabisco)	9
Bran Buds (Kellogg)	8
wheat germ	3
Bran Chex (Ralston)	5
Ralston High Fiber Hot Cereal	5
Corn Bran (Quaker)	5
Weetabix (Weetabix)	4
Bran flakes (any brand)	4
Shredded Wheat n' Bran (Nabisco)	4
Fruit & Fibre (Post)	4

Fiber Content of Cereals

Cereal (1 oz. serving)	dietary fiber (gms)
Cracklin' Oat Bran (Kellogg)	4
Wheatena (Uhlmann)	4
Raisin Bran (Kellogg & Post)	4
bran, unprocessed (3 Tbsp)	4
Oatmeal (Quaker)	2

High-Fiber Low-Calorie Snacks

Snack Food	Calories	fiber (gms)
apple w/ skin (1 med)	81	4
prunes (4)	80	4
fresh strawberries (1 cup)	45	3
raspberries (½ cup)	35	3
pear w/ skin (1 avg)	61	3
apricots (3 med)	51	2
apricots, dried (6 halves)	50	2
banana (1 med)	105	1
peach w/ skin (1 avg)	37	2
pineapple (1 cup)	78	2
figs (3)	68	2
Wasa Fiber Plus crackers (1)	36	3
popcorn (3 cups unbuttered)	75	2
whole wheat toast (1 sl.)	61	2
Ry-Krisp (2 triple crackers)	50	2
broccoli (1 stalk)	24	3
carrot (1 med)	34	2
celery (3 stalks)	21	2

Fiber Content of Vegetables—Greens and Beans

Vegetable (½ c. cooked)	dietary fiber (gms)
peas	4
potato w/ skin (1 med)	3
sweet potato (1 med)	3
corn (cnd)	3
spinach	2
broccoli	2
brussels sprouts	2
turnip	2
zucchini	2
carrots	2

Fiber Content of Legumes

Legumes (½ c. cooked)	dietary fiber (gms)
baked beans (w/ tomato sauce)	9
kidney beans	7
lima and pinto beans	5
split peas	5
lentils	4

Fiber Content of Breads and Pasta

Item	dietary fiber (gms)
whole wheat spaghetti (1 cup cooked)	4
bran muffin (1 med)	3
whole wheat english muffin (1)	3
buckwheat pancakes (2)	3
whole wheat pancakes (2)	3
whole wheat bread (2 slices)	3
whole wheat muffin (1)	2
whole wheat dinner roll (1)	2
whole wheat blueberry muffin (1)	2
brown rice (½ cup cooked)	1

High-Fiber Desserts

Item	dietary fiber (gms)
baked apple stuffed with chopped prunes and dates	6
blackberry pie (⅐ of 9″ pie)	6
stewed fruit compote (prunes, apricots, peaches) ½ cup	4
fresh blackberries (½ cup)	5
whole-wheat banana-nut bread (1 slice)	3
stewed rhubarb (½ cup)	3
fresh strawberries (1 cup)	3

Source: Renneker, M., *Understanding Cancer,* Bull Publishing Co., 1988. Used with permission.

One word of caution, however. When you start adding fiber to your diet, do so gradually. Diving in with large daily portions of fiber-rich foods you used to eat infrequently can have some undesirable side effects that will soon be apparent enough, including flatulence and bloating. And if you suffer from ulcerative colitis, which can sometimes be exacerbated by eating fiber-rich foods, consult with your doctor about the best way to get the fiber you need without aggravating your condition.

Other Benefits of Fruits and Vegetables

It's more than just the fiber in fruits and vegetables that makes eating these foods a valuable part of colorectal cancer prevention. Medical experts believe that a combination of vitamins and nutrients in these foods, often working together, can assist your body's natural functions in fighting off cancer development.

Many of the vitamins that fruits and vegetables contain in abundance are believed to have properties that may help inhibit the initiation stage of colorectal cancer development, when cancer-causing agents prompt normal cells in the large bowel to mutate. Here are some of the benefits:

- Vitamin A (contained in particularly large amounts in carrots, green leafy vegetables, pumpkins, citrus fruits, and melons) fortifies and enhances the body's natural immunity and may also protect cells from carcinogenic assault.
- The B vitamins (particularly in citrus fruits) may increase the anticancer activity of certain enzymes in the bowel that help to dissolve and neutralize carcinogens and move them out of the body.
- Vitamin C boosts the immune system and may even reduce the carcinogenic potency of some foods and other substances lingering in the bowel.
- Vitamins A, C, and E, and beta-carotene (used by your body to produce vitamin A) are also antioxidants, substances that may defend cells from potentially disruptive reactions to the

presence of oxygen. That reaction, called oxidation, can have a harmful effect in the large bowel, damaging DNA and altering genes in a way that may initiate malignant activity.

Vitamin C in particular has been strongly associated with reduced risk of colorectal cancer development. In one study of people with familial polyposis, vitamin C was found to suppress the recurrence of rectal polyps in 80 percent of the patients. Another study discovered that possible carcinogens found in the feces of subjects were no longer seen when daily vitamin C intake was increased (to 400 to 1,000 milligrams—the recommended dietary allowance is only 60 milligrams a day).

There are other substances contained in some vegetables that may be cancer-fighting agents. Beans, as well as rice and seeds (including, but not limited to sunflower, sesame, caraway, and poppy), contain what are called protease inhibitors, that are not digested in the stomach and wind up being passed through the colon where they might help hinder the growth of cancers. Studies performed on groups of people with low rates of colorectal cancer, like Seventh-Day Adventists, have in fact found that diets rich in beans do seem to reduce colorectal cancer development.

Chlorophyll, which is prevalent in raw green vegetables like lettuce, broccoli, and spinach, is active in the large bowel, where it can impede the carcinogenic process. And some researchers are finding that the presence of seaweed in the diet may also reduce the chances of getting colorectal cancer. Rich in fiber, as well as vitamins A, B_{12}, C, and E, seaweed is prevalent in the diet of the Japanese, who, again, have that notably low rate of cancer of the large bowel. Studies conducted on laboratory rats have shown that rats fed large quantities of kelp and kelp extract were less likely to have intestinal tumors than rats that were not fed seaweed. Seaweed products (including hijiki, arame, kombu, nori, and wakame) are available at Asian markets and health food stores and can be introduced into your meals as a subtle garnish in soups and salads. You'll find some good recipes in most macrobiotic cookbooks.

Medical researchers are not certain of the exact mechanisms by which nutrients in fruits and vegetables may inhibit development of cancer of the large bowl. There isn't even final, conclusive evidence that a diet high in produce definitely does have a significant effect. But the signs—and studies—strongly suggest that eating plenty of fruits and vegetables isn't merely sound nutrition, but also a wise risk-reducing enterprise against colorectal cancer.

The important thing, from what we know so far, is not to load up on one kind of food and, especially, on one vitamin supplement. Rather, you should make sure your daily diet includes several portions of a wide variety of fruits and vegetables. That way, you'll receive the full benefit of an array of nutrients that might just help keep you cancer free.

Vitamin D and Calcium

What might account for the wide variations of colorectal cancer incidence in different regions of the United States? Since the 1970s, when medical researchers first began to pay close attention to this phenomenon, investigators have explored the possible roles that vitamin D and calcium may play in colorectal cancer prevention.

Here are the facts: Cancer of the large bowel is more prevalent in the Northeast and significantly less common in the South and Southwest. Colorectal cancer death rates are highest as well in the colder, cloudier portions of the country. And studies also have noted an inverse relation between incidence of cancer of the large bowel and of the skin: Regions with higher rates of skin cancer had lower rates of colorectal cancer.

It was this unusual tendency that led several researchers to explore an intriguing possibility: Could exposure to the sun, the very factor known to be a primary cause of skin cancer, have something to do with discouraging development of colorectal cancer?

The results of studies of vitamin D, one of the chief nutrients the body receives from sunlight, and calcium, a mineral with which vitamin D closely works in the intestine, have led to a wide belief in the medical community that these substances very likely function together to block malignant activity in the large bowel. Calcium cannot be fully absorbed into our bodies from the intestine without the help of vitamin D. The vitamin causes a protein to form in the cells lining the bowel, a protein that passes calcium through the intestinal wall and into the bloodstream. During this process, vitamin D and calcium may actually bind together, also protecting the bowel lining from cancer-causing substances. The presence of these joined nutrients in the colon seems to inhibit cell turnover. And reducing the growth and multiplication of cells along the wall of the intestine can also reduce their vulnerability to carcinogens—and thus their likelihood of becoming mutated and possibly cancerous.

Vitamin D may even work alone to suppress the growth of potentially malignant cells in the intestine. It's been seen with other kinds of cancers; researchers have found that exposing leukemic and melanoma cells to vitamin D in laboratories slows their progress. Unabsorbed calcium, meanwhile, may be doing other cancer-prevention work too, combining with bile acids and fatty acids in the bowel—substances that, as we've seen, can help initiate and promote cancer activity—to flush them out of the body.

Studies attempting to determine the link between vitamin D and calcium and colorectal cancer prevention have been encouraging. For example, in Scandinavia, which has a very high incidence of the disease, areas where people tend to consume large amounts of milk products have lower rates of colorectal cancer. Here in the United States, in a nineteen-year study (conducted by Cedric Garland, Ph.D., and his colleagues at the University of California San Diego School of Medicine) of 2,000 men from Chicago, those whose diets contained the most vitamin D and calcium were almost three times less likely to develop cancer of the large bowel than those whose diets were notably lacking in these nutrients.

Another experiment investigated the effects of increasing the calcium levels of people with a family history of colorectal cancer. These subjects were given large daily doses of a calcium supplement for several months. When examined before the experiment began, many of the subjects showed an excessively rapid buildup of cells lining the bowel wall, an early indication of potential cancerous activity. When they were examined again, after two to three months of receiving the calcium, the cellular activity along the intestinal lining in most of the subjects had largely returned to normal.

In 1989, a report was released that shows some of the strongest evidence of vitamin D's possible role in preventing cancer of the large bowel. In this study, blood samples of 620 people in Maryland were taken to determine their levels of vitamin D. Those with a high concentration of the vitamin had up to an 80 percent reduced risk of developing colorectal cancer.

Sources of Vitamin D

To benefit from the possible cancer-fighting activity of vitamin D and calcium, you need to make sure, of course, that your body receives plentiful amounts of both these nutrients. The set recommended dietary allowance of vitamin D for adults is 200 international units per day; children, teens, pregnant women, and women past menopause usually need more, perhaps as much as 400 international units a day. You can get vitamin D from two major sources: sunlight and diet.

Sunlight. When ultraviolet rays from the sun reach you, they interact with substances in the skin to produce a form of vitamin D. It is then converted in the kidney to become the active nutrient that works together with calcium. Just 5 minutes in the noonday sun while wearing a bathing suit may provide the equivalent of 200 to 300 international units. So exposure to sunlight is a particularly effective way to build your vitamin D intake. It's also an easy way—unless you happen to live in an area that doesn't receive much sunshine. In warmer climates, your bigger concern should be making sure you don't overdo it, spending so much time in the sun without adequate protection that you run the risk of getting skin cancer. But even if you live in the Northeast, for example, you're not doomed to vitamin D deficiency. You do get a certain amount of exposure to ultraviolet sun rays even on overcast days. Plus you don't need a dose of sunshine every single day; the liver can store sunlight-activated vitamin D for later use.

Nevertheless, people living in colder, cloudier regions do have to be on their guard and to rely more heavily on the foods they eat to obtain proper amounts of the vitamin. So do people living in large cities. The tall skyscrapers cast shadows along metropolitan avenues and block the sun, and air pollution blocks ultraviolet rays, cutting the amounts that reach our skin. Colorectal cancer rates in the United States, in fact, tend to be somewhat higher in densely populated areas.

Diet. You will need to be diligent about getting enough vitamin D in your diet, because there isn't a lot of it in much of the food we eat. Some food items, however, do contain significant, even abundant amounts. These include

- *Milk Products.* Now almost always fortified, these are the best dietary sources of vitamin D. One cup of milk contains about one-half the recommended dietary allowance.
- *Red Meat.* Liver and beef are especially high in vitamin D. This is hardly an ideal source, for the purpose of colorectal cancer prevention, because of the high levels of fat and cholesterol also present. Be careful not to rely on red meat too heavily.
- *Eggs.* Again, don't overcompensate and send your cholesterol level soaring.
- *Oily Fish (anchovies and sardines).* Mackerel and salmon are two other kinds of fish high in vitamin D.

As you can see, there are drawbacks to many of these sources of vitamin D—they also happen to be the very sources of substances that can increase your colorectal cancer risk. The best dietary bet is dairy products, including low-fat or nonfat milk, cheese, and yogurt. You should steer away from butter, cream, and sour cream because of their high fat content.

Obstacles to Vitamin D Intake. Although it's not difficult to receive sufficient amounts of vitamin D, plenty of us still aren't getting enough. Older people in particular tend to be vitamin D deficient. Many of the elderly, particularly those who are infirm, don't spend much time at all outdoors. And they often have digestive difficulties that cause them to avoid milk products. Plus, as people age, their skin is not as efficient in producing the nutrient from exposure to ultraviolet rays. Heavily pigmented skin also impedes the production of vitamin D from sunlight.

Sources of Calcium

The current recommended dietary allowance for calcium is 800 milligrams per day, but there's been some discussion about raising that level, and many nutritionists say that, on average, we need closer to 1,200 milligrams per day. Most adult Americans get far less than even the present suggested amount. That doesn't have to be the case, because calcium is common in many of the foods we eat, far more prevalent than vitamin D. These are some of the foods richest in calcium:

- Milk (low-fat milk, besides being lower in fat, also actually contains more calcium than whole milk)
- Cheese (especially Parmesan, ricotta, Swiss, Gruyère, romano, Edam, and cheddar; but because up to three-quarters of the calorie content of some hard cheeses is fat, again, aim for cheeses made with skim or low-fat milk)
- Other dairy products (if you are lactose intolerant, it's likely

you may still be able to tolerate yogurt made from skim
milk)
- Bones (Soft bones in canned sardines and salmon can be
  eaten. Hard bones can be used while simmering soups and
  stews. Add tomatoes, vinegar, or lemon juice; these acids
  will draw out the calcium.)
- Dark green leafy vegetables (spinach, collard greens, kale,
  mustard greens, and turnip greens)
- Broccoli
- Okra
- Blackstrap molasses
- Tofu
- Increasingly, many other kinds of food are being fortified
  with calcium, including bread and enriched flours.

Additional Guidelines

You also have to be careful that the calcium in your body is
used effectively. That means, first off, you have one more good
reason to take advantage of sunny days and to eat foods rich in
vitamin D (several of which, you've undoubtedly noticed, are
also foods rich in calcium). Again, vitamin D is necessary for
calcium absorption, and it's likely these two nutrients need to
work together to give you the full benefit of their colorectal
cancer–inhibiting properties. It's also wise to use less salt and
caffeine, which can disrupt calcium absorption, and to limit the
amount of protein you consume, which often causes calcium to
be eliminated from the body. Or you should compensate for
these foods by adding still extra amounts of calcium to your
diet. Furthermore, if you are taking care to eat enough fiber-rich
foods, then you should also try to consume more calcium, because fiber can hinder the absorption of calcium.

Making calcium and vitamin D a part of your colorectal cancer
risk-reduction program is not hard. It doesn't require doing anything more extraordinary than taking advantage of the sun and
eating the foods rich in these nutrients. The only trick is—and

it's a minor one—to be conscientious about these measures. You can be pretty sure it will be worth it.

Hope for Selenium

It's still rather premature to make solid conclusions about the role of selenium in cancer prevention. But the early evidence has been encouraging. This trace mineral appears in foods like fish (tuna, in particular, but all seafood is a good source), whole grain cereals, Brazil nuts, and organ and muscle meats.

The reason for the recent interest of late in selenium is this: In some animal investigations, selenium supplementation has been shown to inhibit growth of several forms of cancer, including cancer of the large bowel. Meanwhile, initial human studies have found that colorectal cancer patients (and those with other kinds of malignancies) have lower levels of the mineral in the blood than their healthy counterparts.

Thus far, however, researchers know it takes a substantial level of selenium to have any kind of beneficial effect on the laboratory rats being tested. Because the information is still sketchy, most nutritionists and doctors aren't ready to advocate an increased intake of the mineral—but they're eagerly awaiting the results of new, more definitive studies. Even before any categorical evidence arrives, though, as the decade proceeds we may well start seeing more and more foods (like bread and salt) fortified with selenium to help us take advantage of its possible beneficial effects.

A Word About Vitamin and Calcium Supplements and Fiber Pills

There is wide disagreement among medical professionals about the usefulness of supplements. (By medical professionals, we mean licensed physicians and researchers, not the "experts" peddling miracle pills at some alternative health stores who may give you some highly suspect advice.) Most supplements available at reputable stors are manufactured with meticulous care and often do provide valuable nutrients you may not otherwise be getting in sufficient amounts. On the other hand, some products may contain almost toxic levels of certain nutrients. You certainly shouldn't start taking large doses of over-the-counter dietary supplements without first consulting your doctor.

In any event, one thing that most medical professionals agree on is that there is no substitute for the natural way—getting your nutritional requirements by eating the right foods. No studies on the possible cancer-fighting benefits of these substances suggest you should begin consuming inordinately large amounts of them. It also should be mentioned that the National Cancer Institute does not recommend the use of dietary supplements. Once again, a balanced, low-fat, high-fiber diet with plenty of fruits and vegetables should provide you with the nutrients that you need to reduce your chances of developing colorectal cancer, and that may work together in ways we haven't even begun to determine to promote good health.

Aspirin and Colorectal Cancer

According to a report published in December 1991 (*New England Journal of Medicine,* 325: 1593–1596, 1991), aspirin—now commonly used in the prevention of heart attacks and strokes—may also protect against colon cancer. In a large nationwide study headed by Dr. Michael J. Thun of the American Cancer Society, the group of men and women who took sixteen or more aspirins or related drugs (medications like ibuprofen) each month had half the death rate from the disease, compared with the group of those who used the drugs infrequently. The researchers believe aspirin may inhibit the growth of cancer cells already present in the large intestine. Other experts, however, suspect that aspirin users may simply have the benefit of early diagnosis because of the medication's tendency to cause a small amount of intestinal bleeding. In short, although the study is encouraging, it is an early finding and there is still much research to be done. In the meantime, in an interview in the *New York Times* Dr. Thun cautions, "It is premature to recommend taking aspirin . . . to reduce the risk of colon cancer."

Exercise

It is no secret that regular exercise will bring you numerous health benefits. It may well even reduce your risk of colorectal cancer. Although it's hard to tell exactly how, or even if, physical activity itself may help to thwart cancer, people who exercise more do have a proven tendency to be at reduced risk for developing many kinds of malignancies.

Several studies have focused specifically on the possible connection between regular exercise and lower incidence of colorectal cancer. The results have been pretty uniform: People with sedentary jobs and lifestyles have decidedly higher rates of cancer of the large bowel than their more physically active counterparts. And the longer you have foregone a physically active regimen, the greater likelihood you seem to have of eventually developing the disease.

We're a long way from knowing anything specific about the best kind of exercise for reducing risk of colorectal cancer. The day may never come when doctors and physical fitness specialists will be able to design a fitness program for cancer nearly as specific as, say, the kinds of cardiovascular regimes that have been so successful in reducing risk of heart disease. Experts aren't even sure what the connection between exercise and prevention of colorectal cancer may be. Some speculate the benefits come from the overall boost to the immune system that frequent physical activity brings. Others suggest it's not the exercise itself at all, but that physically active people are just more likely to be health conscious, to follow low-fat diets, and to engage in the other kinds of beneficial eating and health practices (including more frequent checkups) that help reduce risk of the disease. It's also reasonable that exercise helps because of where it is performed: Physically active people tend to spend much more time outdoors, where they soak up sunlight, and with it, that invaluable vitamin D.

It doesn't matter if your strength and endurance levels are low to begin with; it's far more important simply that you go out there on a regular basis and "just do it"—after consulting with a physician, of course, if you're over forty, and making sure that you don't *over*do it. Although all our questions can't be answered and certainly no guarantees can be made that x number of laps around the track will reduce your likelihood of colorectal cancer by y percent, engaging in regular exercise is a smart idea indeed, and for many, many reasons even beyond colorectal cancer prevention.

A Word About Tobacco and Alcohol

Smoking and heavy alcohol consumption have been, as we all know, very strongly linked to several kinds of cancer. Their connection to colorectal cancer is much more unclear.

Many studies have attempted to determine whether tobacco smoking will increase the risk of developing cancer of the large bowel the way it does so many other types of cancer. The results have been somewhat contradictory, but the commonly accepted wisdom is that smoking is *not* associated with an increased incidence of colorectal cancer. Several studies, however, have associated smoking with a slightly increased risk of death from colorectal cancer—meaning that if you have cancer of the large bowel and are a smoker, you have a greater likelihood of dying from it. Even here, though, the exact connection is unclear. Does tobacco use cause colorectal cancer to grow and spread faster? Smokers tend to be at a more advanced stage of colorectal cancer than nonsmokers when the disease is first diagnosed. But that may simply be because smokers, being generally less health conscious, are more likely to delay medical care (an assumption that—although it makes sense—has not been conclusively proven).

The alcohol picture is just as murky. Moderate to heavy alcohol consumption has often been suspected to increase at least slightly the risk for colorectal cancer, but the evidence, despite a lot of research, remains conflicting. Some studies have found a link between alcohol consumption and cancer of the large bowel; others have not. Still other studies have found an occasional association; one has determined that when an association exists, it seems to occur even with relatively low alcohol intake, and more likely with beer consumption than other drinks.

The bottom line is this: Although it can't—yet—be said with any certainty that using tobacco or alcohol will increase your chances of getting colorectal cancer, there are so many other excellent reasons to stop smoking and limit your drinking that their possible connection to cancer of the large bowel, or lack thereof, is almost beside the point.

A Word About Asbestos

There are many products, chemicals, and pollutants in our increasingly toxic environment that have been associated with cancer—air pollution, radiation, radon, formaldehyde, pesticides, and toxic waste are only a few, and the list continues to grow. Research has not always pinpointed which specific kinds of cancer are most closely related to exposure to these items. We usually just speak about cancer risk in general. Any cancer, after all, is a serious matter, and one extremely conservative estimate is that up to 5 percent of all cancer deaths result from exposure to some kind of pollution.

That includes exposure to asbestos, a product whose link to higher rates of colorectal cancer specifically, along with several other kinds of cancer, has been determined. Asbestos is contained in many kinds of insulation material that may be used in your home or office, particularly in buildings constructed before 1970. Made up of tiny fibers, it is not hazardous if it remains bonded to other materials. But if the fibers—as they frequently do— become airborne, they can be inhaled or otherwise enter your body, where they can generate dire health problems that may not appear for years.

Asbestos is most closely related to lung, stomach, and esophageal cancer; less often, but still occasionally, to colorectal cancer as well. The real risk for cancer of the large bowel involves people who work with the material, for example, those in the shipbuilding, asbestos mining, and construction professions. But it is possible that living around loose asbestos for a long period of time may also increase your chances of getting colorectal cancer. It's always a good idea, in any event, to have any crumbling asbestos product in your home removed or encapsulated.

If you think asbestos products were used where you live, have an inspection performed by a building contractor or other professional. *It is very dangerous to tamper with asbestos yourself.* A professional will be able to determine if you indeed have a problem and will then be able to remove or encapsulate the material safely.

Questions and Answers

Q: If the experts aren't sure of how, or even whether, eating or avoiding eating certain foods may help prevent cancer, why should I bother to change my diet?

A: Medical professionals are extremely hesitant to make categorical statements. That's particularly true when it comes to the connection between diet and cancer prevention. So many factors are operating simultaneously that it's very hard to isolate the ones that are actually having an influence on cancer development. True, many of us have stocked up on a particular food we heard would prevent some kind of disease, only to find out later that it really had no effect at all. But that's not very likely to happen with the basic dietary recommendations for colorectal cancer prevention, which have been determined after years of investigation and a number of different studies.

The fact is that the medical establishment, reluctant as it is to embrace food fads, does recognize the association between a high-fat, low-fiber diet and a higher incidence of cancer. Organizations like the National Cancer Institute strongly recommend limiting your fat intake and increasing your consumption of fiber, as well as eating a wide assortment of fresh fruits and vegetables and other foods rich in a variety of nutrients. The key thing to remember is that in adding new items to your diet, you must be careful not to throw off your balance by eliminating other nutritious foods (but yes, it is okay to cut out the cake and bacon).

Q: I'm in my fifties and have eaten a high-fat, low-fiber diet all my life. Can changing my eating habits help reduce my chances of getting colorectal cancer at this point?

A: Although you did miss a very good opportunity to start a healthy eating program years ago, there's no reason at all not to begin now. Just as it's never too early to start trying to reduce your risk of colorectal cancer, it's never too late, either. True, some damage may have been already done. But by following a high-fiber, low-fat diet from now on, you at least cut that damage short. And there has been some indication that several of these nutrients actually counteract earlier precancerous activity. Remember the 1989 fiber study discussed on page 66? Polyps that were growing in people who followed the high-fiber regimen were even seen to shrink with some regularity. You still can't exactly count on a dietary change now to counterbalance all the unhealthy practices of a few decades, but it will certainly do a lot more than continuing to eat poorly.

Q: Does anyone ever suggest that people living in cold, cloudy
     parts of the country should actually move to warmer, sun-
     nier regions to help protect themselves against colorectal
     cancer?

A: Certainly no reasonable medical professional would say you
     have to go to such extremes. While a study of people who've
     moved from colder climates to sunnier ones does show a
     somewhat reduced incidence of colorectal cancer, you are
     hardly doomed if you remain up north. Getting enough
     vitamin D is entirely possible, even in consistently overcast
     areas. In the first place, it hardly requires *constant* exposure
     to the sun (that's dangerous anyway, putting you at greatly
     increased risk of skin cancer). And living in Hartford, Con-
     necticut, for instance, isn't exactly like being on the planet
     Pluto. While you do have to take greater care than you
     would living in Santa Monica, for example, there is more
     than just the occasional sunny day practically anywhere you
     make your home; take advantage of them. Get the sunshine
     you can and be sure to supplement your diet with regular
     helpings of those foods, particularly low-fat milk products,
     that are good sources of vitamin D.

5

The Symptoms

SELF-TEST

Have you recently experienced

		Score
1.	Rectal bleeding?	_____
2.	Anemia?	_____
3.	Diarrhea that has persisted for two weeks or more?	_____
4.	Constipation that has persisted for two weeks or more?	_____
5.	Alternating diarrhea and constipation?	_____
6.	An urgent desire to go to the bathroom when there is no need?	_____
7.	Repeated bowel movements in which the stool was very thin in diameter?	_____

8. Stools that are jet-black or blood-red in color? _____
9. Abdominal cramps or pain? _____
10. Unexplained gradual weight loss or loss of
    appetite? _____
11. Unexplained general weakness or fatigue? _____
12. Unexplained fever? _____
13. Unexplained palpable lump in the abdominal
    area? _____
14. Enlargement of the liver? _____
15. Unexplained lower back pain? _____
16. Unusual bladder symptoms? _____

Any of these conditions may be a sign that you have colorectal cancer. In this chapter, we'll discuss exactly what these symptoms may mean, why they do not necessarily indicate the presence of cancer itself, and why, nevertheless, it's vital to follow up on any and all of them just to make sure.

What to Watch For

Throughout this book so far, we've discussed the factors—physical, hereditary, and environmental—that may make you vulnerable to developing colorectal cancer. You've seen how important it is to receive regular screenings if you are in a high-risk group. But there are other portentous indications that testing for cancer of the large bowel is necessary. Before we discuss the various diagnostic exams for colorectal cancer, let's take a look at the symptoms of the disease.

One fact above all must be emphasized: *You certainly shouldn't wait until these symptoms develop before you are examined.* They are often signs, after all, that a malignancy has already started to grow, and it's obviously preferable to detect the problem earlier, which, as we'll see, is quite likely to happen if you follow a regular screening program.

The signs indicating the possible presence of cancer in the large bowel actually are frustratingly nonspecific. Rather than being clear signals exclusively of the presence of cancer, many of these symptoms are often related to other, entirely different ailments as well. The symptoms, in fact, much more frequently are manifestations of a condition far less serious than cancer. But you still must treat them very, very seriously. If any of these symptoms persists for more than two weeks, it's vital—particularly if you are over forty or if your health or family background place you at high risk for the disease—that you talk to your doctor, so the possibility of cancer of the large bowel can be ruled out . . . or perhaps confirmed.

Another reason why you must not rely entirely on the appearance of symptoms, in addition to the fact that they so often indicate some other ailment, is that cancer may be present in the colon or rectum literally for years without producing any signs or warnings at all, all the while continuing to grow. That's worth saying again: *Colorectal cancer may be asymptomatic for years*.

Generally, the symptoms that do appear are related to the size and location of the malignancy. Cancers growing in the rectum or sigmoid colon are much more likely to be symptomatic early on in the course of the disease; tumors growing in the cecum or ascending colon, on the other hand, because they are apt to remain close to the bowel wall and don't obstruct the interior, will often remain silent for a long time. But because the warning signs tend to appear the further along a malignancy has developed, asymptomatic persons are still usually more likely to be at an earlier stage of the disease and thus generally have a more favorable prognosis. Another important thing to know is that the duration of a symptom, once it has persisted for two weeks or more, usually has nothing to do with the extent of the cancer, or even the likelihood that a malignancy exists.

These introductory remarks made, let's go through the symptoms of colorectal cancer, one by one, and see what they may indicate.

Bleeding

The appearance of blood is often the first symptom of colorectal cancer that is noticed; it may be caused by malignancies growing virtually anywhere in the large bowel. Most bowel cancers produce at least small amounts of blood. Oftentimes a malignant or benign polyp, particularly if it reaches into the lumen (bowel interior), will bleed because it gets jostled and irritated by the stool coming down the intestinal path. Villous adenomas—a type of polyp less common but more often cancerous than tubular adenomas—also bleed more frequently and can cause mucus to be excreted in the stool as well.

Because the bowel is wider in the right colon, malignancies growing there have room to become large enough to cause internal bleeding. In the narrower left colon, a tumor is more likely to cause at least a partial blockage of the intestine, which also may result in bleeding. And malignancies developing in the rectum, because they may grow in the reservoir area where feces are held before being discharged, are especially likely to produce bloody stools.

If an ample enough amount of blood is involved, you'll frequently see it when you go to the bathroom. What you will notice is often the appearance of fairly bright red blood on the surface or mixed in with the stool, or the appearance of blood on the toilet paper. Although the bleeding may be acute, oftentimes only a microscopic amount of blood is involved, far too little for you to notice. That's why occult (hidden) blood tests are a regular part of colorectal cancer screening.

Of course, the appearance of blood is also—and more commonly—caused not by colorectal cancer, but by hemorrhoids. Too often, however, that's the diagnosis a person or his or her doctor will automatically make, neglecting to bother with any follow-up tests. It's crucial, no matter what your doctor says, that the possibility of colorectal cancer be at least considered and explored thoroughly.

Iron-Deficiency Anemia

This may be the result of the slow, frequent, but often imperceptible internal bleeding that often results from a tumor's presence in the cecum or ascending colon. While blood loss can also occur with malignancies in the rectum and sigmoid colon, cancer in these parts of the bowels is not likely to cause anemia.

Unexplained anemia is often a good indication there may be trouble in your large bowel. Once again, however, many patients and doctors alike are too prone to explain away this warning. In older people, we frequently assume it is simply another aspect of aging. And that is often true. Nevertheless, *any* unexplained iron-deficiency anemia, particularly among older persons and particularly when it accompanies signs of blood in the stool, requires a thorough evaluation by a doctor.

Change in Bowel Habits

Diarrhea, constipation, or other changes in bowel habits related to the presence of colorectal cancer or to precursors of the disease often appear intermittently and may have alternating active and inactive phases. But they do tend to persist over a period of time, unlike when they're merely caused by a particular unfortunate encounter with, say, unfiltered water. If you experience any of the following symptoms, even sporadically, over several weeks, and they appear unrelated either to anything you may have eaten or drunk or to a virus you may have been battling, talk to your doctor, for they could be an indication of possible benign polyps or malignancies growing in the large bowel:

Diarrhea. Tumors in the rectum commonly cause diarrhea, which is often, although not always, streaked with blood. Sometimes the diarrhea is quite real. But you may also frequently feel a strong, even overwhelming and painful urge to defecate when there is no need, causing you to make repeated seemingly necessary trips to the bathroom that wind up being unsuccessful or incomplete. That's because the malignancy growing in the rectal wall may give the sensation of being a bowel movement that has not been evacuated.

Constipation. Malignancies growing in the narrower, left part of the colon can become large enough to encircle the entire bowel wall, causing partial intestinal blockage. The result may be increasing constipation, frequently accompanied by distension, bloating, and gas. A tumor extending out from the rectal wall may cause constipation as well, or alternating constipation and diarrhea, by obstructing the flow of feces. Chronic constipation, incidentally, may also be a sign of other forms of cancer, including cancer of the kidney and the ovaries.

Change in Stool Size. Blockage by growing tumors of the left colon or rectum may cause stools much narrower in diameter than normal to form. It's not abnormal occasionally to have thin, even reedy bowel movements. But if you notice this feature during several—or especially all—of your trips to the bathroom over a period of a couple weeks, you should discuss this, and other unusual bowel habits, with your doctor.

Change in Stool Color. Blood in the feces may be responsible for turning the stool jet black in color. You may even have blood red stools, a sure sign of rectal bleeding, and that means you should see your doctor at once for a complete exam.

Abdominal Pain

Abdominal pain is a common symptom of cancerous tumors that grow throughout the large bowel. In addition to causing internal bleeding, malignancies in the cecum or ascending colon may grow large enough to cause you to feel pain in the right abdomen. The bowel obstruction resulting from tumors growing around the walls of the transverse or descending colon often produces intermittent crampy or gaseous pain. This discomfort is frequently and particularly felt after meals, worsened by eating and relieved upon the passage of gas and feces. Cancers in the sigmoid colon and rectum may also result in your feeling significant pain accompanied by a chronic sensation of fullness. In addition, perforation of the bowel by a growing tumor may be the cause of abdominal pain.

Generally, the larger the tumors in your colon and rectum have grown, the more likely you are to experience abdominal pain. Although, as with the other symptoms we've discussed, significant abdominal discomfort is often entirely unrelated to colorectal cancer, you should consider it to be a sign of a condition that requires prompt attention and so should report it to a doctor right away.

Weight Loss and Loss of Appetite

Because colorectal cancer disrupts the normal functions of your digestive system, gradual and unexplained weight loss or long-term loss of appetite may follow. Tumors growing on the bowel wall can interfere with the intestine's ability to absorb water, minerals, and remaining nutrients into your bloodstream and lymph nodes, depriving your body of these vital materials and resulting in your losing weight in a most undesired manner. And the vague dis-ease and discomfort you may experience can work to curb your appetite without your being aware of the cause. Your doctor can help you determine whether the possibility of cancer should be considered and tests to make a definite determination scheduled.

Weakness and Fever

Relatively advanced cancers of the large bowel may cause you to run a high temperature over a period of time and experience unusual paleness and chronic general fatigue. These symptoms, too, can be indications of any number of illnesses besides colorectal cancer. Nevertheless, if unexplained fever and weakness persist, and particularly if you've experienced any of the other symptoms in the past or presently experience them, you should see a physician for a thorough general physical examination that will help to narrow down their probable cause.

Mass or Lump

The discovery of a mass that you can feel in the abdominal area is not the early indication of cancer that a palpable lump in the breast may be. Rather, it is a possible late indication of the presence of a large tumor in the colon, or in the liver, ovaries, or pancreas. That would mean cancer at an advanced stage and should be reported right away to your doctor.

Enlargement of the Liver, Pain in the Lower Back or Posterior, and Bladder Symptoms

These symptoms, particularly when persistent, may indicate grave extension of malignant tumors through the bowel wall or the spread of cancer from the bowel to other regions, including the liver or bladder; the prostate for men; and the cervix, ovaries, or uterus for women. If cancer is indeed the cause, they are often signs that the disease is at an advanced stage.

But, once again, these could also be symptoms of one of a number of other conditions entirely unrelated to malignant activity. Back and posterior pain, of course, can be nothing more than the aftereffects of a rigorous touch football game or horseback outing, although, to be sure, a chronic discomfort hitherto nonexistent is reason for greater concern. An enlarged liver will frequently be palpable in the upper right abdominal area and is always a symptom to take seriously. So are unusual bladder symptoms, including abnormalities like the presence of blood or pus in the urine and an increased need to urinate, especially at night. Without consulting a physician, however, there's no accurate way of narrowing down the likely cause of any of these symptoms, so it is crucial to talk to your doctor to ascertain what steps should be taken in diagnosing the problem.

The Bottom Line

If you think all these symptoms seem terribly nonspecific—that none of them points with certainty to colorectal cancer—then you understand correctly. There really aren't any physical signs unique to colorectal cancer. Consider this: About 12 percent of all people report in their physical examinations that they recently experienced a change in bowel habits. Yet very few of them are found to have colorectal cancer. Approximately 11 percent complain of abdominal pain, but the great majority of them are free of any malignancy. And for only about 8 percent of the people who suffer from rectal bleeding is that symptom indeed related to cancer of the large bowel.

These should be comforting statistics—but don't let them comfort you so excessively or unwisely that your diligence falters. The unfortunate thing is that in the relatively small percentage of cases where the symptoms *are* caused by colorectal cancer, they are so often incorrectly diagnosed and confused with very minor ailments and even with the everyday vagaries of life. That's bad news, but only if we—and our doctors—go right ahead and assume the best without thinking or checking further.

The good news, however, is that if you and your physician *do* follow through, you're likely to find out that the condition you are suffering from is probably something other than, and something much less serious than, cancer. And you'll know for sure.

Same Symptoms, Different Ailments

Let's take a quick look at some of the most common ailments and conditions that share some of these same symptoms. This information isn't meant to reassure you falsely. It will simply further show you that an abdominal cramp or some rectal bleeding does not inevitably, or even usually, mean a diagnosis of cancer. Just be sure you don't use this information to close your

eyes and shrug off nagging and persistent warning signs. It can't
be said often enough: *Don't fear that these symptoms mean the
worst, but certainly don't assume they mean nothing, or nothing
much.* Report them to your physician, get a general physical
exam or a specific examination of the colon and rectum as the
situation warrants, if only to find out that you merely suffer
from one of the following conditions.

Hemorrhoids

It's true that hemorrhoids are the most frequent cause of rectal
bleeding. The problem, again, is when they're automatically assumed to be the culprit, allowing the possibility of cancer or
other serious intestinal disorders to be dangerously overlooked.

The blood from hemorrhoids is usually bright red and found
dripping into the toilet bowl, on the surface of the stool, or on
the toilet paper. Hemorrhoids also frequently cause itching and
other anal discomfort. A person who discovers blood upon a
trip to the bathroom, especially if it has been accompanied by
that proverbial "pain and itch," should not get too scared and
should be heartened by the likelihood it's all simply caused by
hemorrhoids. Nevertheless, the bleeding, even if it is accompanied by pain and itching, must be investigated further. No
matter how much you want to believe it, don't let a lazy doctor
shrug off this warning sign without any testing whatsoever.
That's the time for a second opinion. And perhaps it's also time
you consider taking your business elsewhere—your business
being, after all, your continued good health—to a meticulous
physician who knows to take warning signs like this, whatever
the likelihood that no grave problem exists, very, very seriously.

Virus

Diarrhea or constipation is almost always just a short-lived
and occasional unpleasant fact of life. It's when they're not short
lived and not occasional that they have a greater likelihood of

indicating something more serious. Still, attacks that last several days are usually caused by influenza or an intestinal virus. If these conditions are accompanied by other typical symptoms of flu or viral infection and go away around the same time as the illness does, then there's usually no need at all for any follow-up. If, however, diarrhea or constipation linger or alternate with each other for more than two or three weeks or if they seem to be entirely unrelated to illness or anything you may have eaten, and even if they occur intermittently but over a longer period of time, these may well be indications that specific testing for the possible presence of a malignancy in the large bowel is advisable.

Inflammatory Bowel Disease

Chronic ulcerative colitis and Crohn's disease commonly produce symptoms strikingly similar to those of colorectal cancer, including frequent rectal bleeding, diarrhea, abdominal pain and cramping, and even fever and weight loss. In fact, inflammatory bowel disease is diagnosed using most of the same screening methods as those used to detect cancer of the large bowel. Because the disease is also a serious, long-term condition, one that requires regular monitoring and sometimes medication, and because it has a chance of eventually leading to colorectal cancer, the symptoms listed above must not be ignored.

Irritable Bowel Syndrome

Also known by the erroneous term "spastic colon," irritable bowel syndrome is not a disease per se, but rather what's considered a functional abnormality. It is usually provoked by stress, perhaps even more by certain foods and beverages (like strong spices, raw fruit and vegetables, coffee, and alcoholic drinks), and, whatever its status as a "mere" abnormality, the symptoms and discomfort are quite real. These include sharp, stabbing abdominal pain or perhaps a deep dull ache, as well as abnormal bowel functions, constipation more commonly than diarrhea. From long, unpleasant experience, most people with spastic colon are well aware they suffer from this condition. If you are one of them and you experience any of these warning signs over an unusually extended period of time, you should first consider if, indeed, you have recently undergone any emotional pressure or turmoil, or perhaps had a questionable eating experience. But if the symptoms continue or appear unrelated to stress or food, you should see your doctor. And if you never previously had a spastic bowel episode, you certainly should report to a doctor when these warning signs appear.

Diverticular Disease

As many as one-third of all Americans over forty-five, and two-thirds over sixty, experience diverticular disease. Like colorectal cancer, it is especially prevalent in parts of the world where the diet tends to be low in fiber. Diverticular disease involves the formation of small pockets, or outpouchings, called *diverticula* in the bowel wall. Usually, this is entirely harmless and produces no symptoms. But occasionally the diverticula may become inflamed, causing alternating bouts of diarrhea and constipation (or other abnormal bowel habits), pain in the lower abdomen, fever, and the appearance of blood (especially dark, as opposed to red, blood) in the stool. If you experience any of these symptoms and are of an age where diverticular disease is likely, you should not merely assume that to be the cause, but rather you should have it checked by your doctor. Of course, by that age you should already be receiving regular exams of the colon interior that will indicate the presence of these pockets.

Other Obstructions of the Bowel

Malignant tumors or benign polyps are not the only things that can cause a narrowing of the large intestine. Scarring and thickening of the bowel wall, caused by such conditions as diverticular, Crohn's disease, and radiation enterocolitis, as well as strictures resulting from ulcerative colitis, may obstruct passage of waste material and can result in your having bowel movements that are regularly, perhaps always, thin. There's really no way of knowing what's causing the obstruction without a peek inside the colon, so it's a good idea to undergo an endoscopic exam to rule out the possibility of cancer.

Appendicitis

Yes, it's possible that you can mistake pain caused by acute appendicitis for a possible warning sign of colorectal cancer. Usually, however, you should be able to tell the difference. Appendicitis is signaled by a very distinctive, sudden, and sharp pain that occurs specifically in the lower right-hand abdominal area. Whatever the cause, this is obviously a very serious warning sign that demands immediate medical attention.

Occasionally, however, particularly among older people, the appendicitis may have actually been triggered by the presence of cancer in the cecum. Many doctors recommend, therefore, that senior citizen appendicitis patients be endoscopically examined after a suitable recovery period.

Questions and Answers

Q: Okay, so constipation is a symptom of colorectal cancer. But can it also *cause* colorectal cancer?

A: In a recent film comedy, there's a scene where two advertising executives unveil a new promotional pitch for a brand of laxative: "Use our product; if you don't, you'll get cancer." Actually, there's no conclusive evidence whatsoever that such a direct link exists. On the other hand, when you are constipated, undigested food lingers in the bowel for longer periods and, yes, any carcinogenic material you may have consumed has a little more time to affect cells in the colon and rectum. One reason, in fact, why fiber is suspected of being so beneficial in colorectal cancer prevention is because it speeds up digestion and sends waste material—and the harmful substances contained within—flowing through the large intestine quickly. That doesn't mean you should go start swallowing laxatives at the first sign of "irregularity." What's far more important is what you eat in the first place. The occasional bout of constipation has extremely little effect on your chances of developing cancer and usually is nothing more than an inconvenience. Your best bet for chronic constipation (once you've had exams to rule out colorectal cancer or other possibly serious causes) is not to rely on laxatives, which may irritate the bowel if taken too often, but to handle it naturally, gradually increasing your fiber intake by eating an assortment of fiber-rich foods.

Q: I'm sixty-three and have had diverticular disease for several years. I've even, in the past, experienced occasional inflammation, with diarrhea, abdominal pain, bleeding, and the like. Now I'm experiencing these symptoms again. How do I know they're caused by inflammation of those outpockets and not by cancer?

A: You *don't* know for sure, unless—you guessed it—you have a complete examination of the large bowel. Because inflammation of the diverticula itself merits attention, and because you're at an age when colorectal cancer is most common, it's a decidedly wise idea to make that appointment with your doctor.

Q: I recently found out I'm anemic and have also been experiencing some irregular bowel habits. I took one of those occult blood tests and the results came out negative. But my diarrhea and constipation persist. Should I still be concerned?

A: One of the reasons, as we'll discuss in the next chapter, why occult blood tests are a somewhat controversial screening measure is because they frequently give "false negative" results. In other words, the test may indicate that there's no blood in the stool even when there really is a problem. As a result, people who should be examined further are lulled into a false sense of security and wind up seeking no further testing or treatment until much later—even too late. Because you continue to experience other warning signs, you are right to be concerned. Do make sure you continue exploring the cause of these symptoms. Get another test, and, perhaps, another medical opinion.

Q: If I experience any of the symptoms listed here, does that automatically mean I have to have a full set of colon and rectum examinations?

A: No. Because several of these symptoms indicate the likelihood of some significant disorder of the large bowel, an exam of the bowel interior will not only rule out the possibility of cancer but will also help the doctor diagnose the condition that actually exists. But many of the other symptoms—weakness, fever, and weight loss—may be caused by any number of ailments, and a consultation with the doctor can narrow down the possibilities. It's not necessary at all in those cases to start right away with the rectal and colon probes. The important thing when you realize you have any of these symptoms is to share this information with a doctor. Then the two of you together can plot the proper course of action.

6

Screening: For Diagnosis, Early Detection, and Prevention

The Second Line of Defense

Yes, you should be examined thoroughly if you have any of the warning signs of colorectal cancer. But once again it must be said: That's hardly the only occasion when it greatly behooves you to be tested. If following the lifestyle practices we've discussed constitutes the primary defense against colorectal cancer, a regular screening program for those at risk of the disease, even when you don't experience any symptoms at all, is nothing less than the second level of defense. It is an essential element of colorectal cancer prevention.

Just how effective can screening be? There's no way to quantify how often regular screening actually prevents cancer. Benign polyps are removed without our knowing for certain whether they would have ultimately become malignant or not. But we do know this: Malignant tumors may grow for years in the bowel without causing any symptoms. And several routine tests that are readily available, relatively inexpensive, and not terribly inconvenient can detect even the smallest benign growths in the colon or rectum, sometimes years before you'd otherwise know you have them.

Numerous studies confirm this. One investigation has estimated that up to 95 percent of all early-stage cancers can be found through early detection programs. This is twice the number detectable through conventional experience. Other research strongly suggests that the detection of colorectal cancer before the onset of symptoms increases the chances of being cured. And still other investigations have found that the death rate from colorectal cancer was far lower among those subjects who were screened regularly. In one study 90 percent survived 15 years or longer, many more than those colorectal cancer patients who had not been routinely examined.

That doesn't mean we all constantly need to be on the examining table. A practical, effective screening program utilizing a combination of these diagnostic exams, based on your particular health and family background—a program that reduces your risk of colorectal cancer and increases your chances for detecting any malignancy in an early stage—actually demands very little of your time and money, considering the benefits. You begin by consulting your family doctor, who will determine the kinds of screening procedures you should undergo and the regularity with which you ought to have them conducted. General practitioners are well qualified to perform several of these exams themselves. For procedures that are outside your physician's area of expertise, he or she should be able to refer you to a specialist, generally a gastroenterologist, who is trained in the care of conditions of the whole gastrointestinal tract, or a proctologist, who treats diseases of the colon and rectum. A radiologist is called on to conduct the X-ray exams that are sometimes a part of the screening process.

Before we discuss the recommended colorectal cancer screening programs for different risk groups, let's take a look at the exams and procedures most commonly used in the detection of the disease.

Fecal Occult Blood Test

Rectal bleeding, as we've seen, may indicate the presence of a cancerous tumor in the colon or rectum. It may also, just as important, denote a benign polyp that could eventually become malignant. Oftentimes, the blood is easily noticeable when you go to the bathroom, appearing in the stool, dripping into the toilet bowl, or appearing on the toilet tissue. But frequently, only microscopic amounts of blood are secreted by a malignancy and are impossible to observe visually. Fecal occult blood tests are used to detect the presence of this hidden, or occult, blood in the stool.

This screening exam involves a simple chemical testing of the stool. Generally, you are asked to prepare a set of slides at home by placing several small stool samples on pieces of chemically treated paper.

Your doctor will give you specific instructions for the test. Most patients are told to begin a modified diet at least 24 to 48 hours before the first sample is taken. That commonly means staying clear of red meat, vitamin C, iron supplements, and aspirin, all of which may interfere with accurate test results. In addition, it's often recommended to eat plenty of high-fiber foods, because the fiber can stimulate the bleeding of polyps or malignancies. While remaining on this diet, it's likely you'll be asked to collect two separate stool samples, from two different trips to the bathroom, over each of the following three days. You then return these samples, usually by mail, to the doctor for laboratory analysis. The cost of this exam is very low and you'll get the results quickly.

In addition to these laboratory-evaluated tests, there are several varieties of do-it-yourself kits that test for fecal occult blood available at many pharmacies. These at-home tests usually cost no more than $5 and tend to come in three different forms: (1) a slide and developing solution, (2) chemically permeated paper to drop into the toilet bowl after you've gone to the bathroom, and (3) specially prepared wipes. The specifics differ depending on the kit used, but in most cases a color change on the paper should indicate if even microscopic amounts of blood are present in the stool.

If the results of any fecal blood test are positive, meaning the presence of blood is indicated, then you must follow up with further screening by your doctor to determine the source of the bleeding.

The Results Are Controversial

And therein lies part of the problem—and the controversy—of the effectiveness of this screening method. Although fecal blood tests are simple, quick, and inexpensive, the information derived from them can be vague and even downright misleading—and that can be dangerous. A positive blood test does not necessarily, or even usually, mean cancer; likewise, a negative test, indicating an absence of blood, does not necessarily mean you are free of any malignancies in your colon or rectum. The reason why, in fact, stool samples are taken over several days is to increase the likelihood that bleeding will be detected. But fecal blood tests still miss a substantial number of cases or provide contradictory results that require more accurate screening measures to clarify.

False positive results are more common than false negatives. Blood in the stools, as we've seen, can come from many sources other than benign or malignant tumors. Hemorrhoids are the most common culprits, but bleeding can also be caused by diverticular disease, inflammatory bowel disease, or even merely consumption of the foods and substances (like red meat or aspirin) that you're told to avoid while taking the exam.

False negative results occur simply when malignancies in the large bowel don't happen to bleed during the period you take the test. That's not unusual: As we've seen, some cancers in the colon and rectum cause bleeding only intermittently and others don't bleed at all. Larger polyps and those growing in the right side of the colon are more likely to bleed and are thus more likely to be detected through this test. The high-fiber diet you're encouraged to eat during the testing period is meant to stimulate bleeding, but often it does not. The stool sample, meanwhile, may not have even come in contact with a tumor growing in the left side of the colon, and thus might not mix with any blood it excretes.

The statistics for false positive and false negative readings from fecal occult blood tests are alarming. One study found that just 40 to 50 percent of those people whose tests were positive had any adenomatous growth in the large bowel whatsoever, 12 percent of them actually had cancer, and the rest had benign polyps. Other research has suggested that only 5 to 10 percent of people with positive test results turn out to have a malignancy. Furthermore, a positive blood test is less likely to signify cancer or the presence of a polyp in a younger person. One review concluded that a forty-year-old whose test is positive has about a 20 percent chance of having a polyp or malignancy; in a fifty-year-old the chances increase to 50 percent. Furthermore, on the false negative side, several studies of people with colorectal cancer showed that 20 to 30 percent of them received negative fecal blood results and only one-third of those with benign polyps tested positive.

You can see how the ramifications of inaccurate results can be serious. False positive tests mean further testing that is costly, inconvenient, not very pleasant, and most often unnecessary. The consequences of false negative tests are even more perilous. Wrongly reassured that you are cancer free, you may avoid seeking the medical attention and treatment you need, and may even disregard further symptoms and warning signs of the disease.

Because of this high degree of inaccuracy, many experts are

unconvinced of the overall advantages of stool blood testing as a screening measure for colorectal cancer. Some go even further. Several study groups, including one organized by the National Cancer Institute, consider the test altogether inadequate, maintaining that the drawbacks wind up outweighing the benefits.

Others, however, continue to contend that fecal blood testing has an important role to play. Dr. David Eddy, an adviser on screening tests to both the American Cancer Society and the National Cancer Institute, used a mathematical model to determine the test's usefulness. Because the test can indicate the presence of a small polyp that could eventually become malignant if not removed, Eddy concluded that people over forty who take the test annually decrease their chances of ever getting colorectal cancer by 15 percent. And, because it can detect cancer in an early, highly treatable stage (remember that bleeding is often the first symptom of a large bowel malignancy), an annual test can decrease the chances of dying from the disease by up to 40 percent.

The American Cancer Society resolutely endorses the use of fecal blood testing as part of an overall screening program that includes the other tests we are about to discuss.

It is recommended you take the fecal blood test annually, even if you have no symptoms, once you reach fifty.

What you need to keep in mind is that you should not panic if the results are positive, nor should you be overly confident if they are negative.

Even with a positive reading, there's still a good chance that you do not have cancer. Again, what you may have is a potentially threatening polyp that, once detected through this screening, can be removed. You will need to have follow-up tests to determine the exact cause of the bleeding, especially if you are over fifty, when the likelihood of cancer is higher.

Similarly, you must not ignore persistent warning signs even if your test was negative, particularly if you are in a high-risk group. Report these symptoms to your doctor and be sure you continue to be on your guard and follow an appropriate regular colorectal cancer screening regime.

Digital Rectal Exam

This quick, simple, and utterly routine test is commonly performed by a doctor as part of a general physical examination. The physician inserts a gloved, well-lubricated finger into the rectum, feeling for abnormalities in the rectal wall, particularly for unusually firm areas that may signify polyps or malignant tumors (for male patients, the prostate is also checked). At the same time, the doctor may visually examine the anal area for any irregularities and may also collect a small stool sample for an occult blood test.

The digital rectal exam takes only seconds to perform and it's entirely painless, safe, and sanitary, albeit somewhat embarrassing. Many doctors will attempt to make it easier by distracting you as they perform the procedure, engaging in some routine conversation while they furtively prepare and guide you into the position. If you miss that distinctive snap of rubber as the physician slips glove over hand, you may not even realize what's happening until the rectal exam is under way, removing the jittery anticipation that constitutes the only difficult part of this test.

While it continues to be a valuable screening exam for malignancies in the lower rectum—any malignant tumor growing within 3 or so inches of the anus can usually be felt—the digital exam is not as reliable a method for detecting colorectal cancer as it has been in the past. That's because over the past several years there has been an increasing incidence of cancer developing further up the colon. Currently, this method can detect only about 10 to 15 percent of all large bowel cancers. So receiving a digital rectal exam alone does not mean you have been completely or sufficiently screened for all possible malignancies.

Nevertheless, it should continue to be a regular part of your physical exam, even if you are not in a high-risk group for colorectal cancer and have not displayed any symptoms of the disease. The American Cancer Society recommends that everyone forty years and over take this test annually.

A Word About Self-Examination

The word is Don't. Aside from at-home fecal occult blood tests, the pros and cons of which we've already discussed, there's no equivalent in colorectal cancer for the self-exam that's a regular and integral part of breast cancer screening and prevention. Still, you may have come across, while reading other literature, some discussion and instructions for examining your own anus and rectum. *Be very wary.* This kind of self-examination is no substitute at all for screening by a physician, and it is rarely recommended by reputable doctors and medical organizations. Screening and diagnosis of colorectal cancer is far too serious, complicated, and intricate a matter to leave in our own hands, as it were. And because self-palpation is indeed rather unsavory, as well as awkward and even prone to causing infection if not performed under sanitary conditions, you'll find it much simpler, and so much wiser, to go to a physician who has the experience and knowledge to do the job right.

Endoscopy

Endoscopy is a general term referring to any examination of the inside of the body using optical instruments to look at hollow organs or body cavities. It plays a major role in the detection—and even prevention—of colorectal cancer. There are several different endoscopic exams used in the screening of this disease. *Sigmoidoscopy,* also called *proctosigmoidoscopy* or simply *proc-*

toscopy, is an examination of the lower portion of the large bowel; _colonoscopy_ is an examination of the entire large bowel. The kind of test performed depends on several factors, including the symptoms you may be experiencing, the growths or other abnormalities revealed in prior screening tests, and even the kind of training your physician has received.

Rigid Sigmoidoscopy

This is the proctoscopic exam that gives proctoscopic exams a bad name. Until recently, it was the only option for inspecting the large bowel that didn't involve great time, expense, and even a hospital stay. The rigid sigmoidoscopy is still in use, and in some circumstances, it may be perfectly adequate or even the wisest exam option. It is also rather unpleasant. Whether the procedure is downright painful or merely uncomfortable and embarrassing is really just a matter of semantics. Fortunately, however, it is relatively cheap, entirely safe, and—thankfully—relatively brief.

The procedure is usually performed right in your doctor's examination room. Before your appointment, you will have undergone either minimal or extensive bowel preparation, depending on the doctor's recommendation. Many physicians believe a simple phosphosoda enema, purchased over the counter and taken at home 1 or 2 hours before the exam will suffice; others will instruct you to follow a liquid diet or to fast altogether for several hours, and also to take an enema or suppository. Once you are at the doctor's office, you may be given another enema to make sure your lower bowel is clear. Then, you'll be instructed to lie either face down in a kneeling position, draped over the exam table with your buttocks in the air, or on your side with knees bent. The doctor will usually give a digital rectal exam immediately before commencing with the sigmoidoscopy itself.

The rigid scope is a well-lubricated, narrow, essentially hollow tube about 10 inches long with a magnified viewing system. One end, encircled with a fiberoptic ring for lighting, is inserted in the anus, and is slowly—and as delicately as possible—passed into the rectum and sigmoid colon. The doctor is able to peer through the other end, the light illuminating the dark recesses of the bowel, to examine the intestinal wall for any growths or other abnormalities. The scope is also equipped with a smaller channel that allows air to be pumped through. This will expand the bowel walls (although deft physicians won't always need to) both to make it easier for the scope to pass and to make the crevices of the walls, which may be obscured by folds or mucus, more visible (experienced physicians, however, don't always have to "insufflate," or introduce air, when they use the rigid scope). The doctor can carefully inspect about 6 to 8 inches past the anus with the rigid scope. Because of the air being puffed into the intestine and because of the presence of the instrument itself, you may feel an urge to defecate during the exam. And you won't be able to help some flatulence escaping around the instrument; don't even try to control it. Throughout the exam, you should keep breathing deeply and slowly to help relax the abdominal muscles. The procedure itself is relatively brief, in experienced hands usually taking less than 5 minutes. Rigid sigmoidoscopy is a relatively inexpensive exam—customarily costing in the range of $70 to $150—and often covered by health insurance.

So it's quick, safe, and fairly cheap—what's the drawback? In the first place, the usefulness of this screening exam is severely compromised by the fact that it's so unpleasant. It's not unusual for many, even those who are well aware of their risk of colorectal cancer, to shy away from this procedure. Even many physicians in the field admit that they too are lax about receiving the exam themselves.

The effectiveness of rigid sigmoidoscopy is also limited by the relatively short length of the bowel that can be examined. Only about 20 to 25 percent of colorectal cancers develop in the area of the bowel reachable by the rigid scope. And again, because malignancies developing farther up the bowel are becoming more prevalent, the usefulness of this procedure has declined slightly in recent years.

And if not altogether obsolete, its use is declining as greater numbers of doctors are trained in the use of the more thorough and far less unpleasant flexible sigmoidoscopes. What keeps the rigid scope in use? To begin with, it's a less costly test. Also, many doctors remain untrained in the newer procedure and don't have the instruments. And in many cases, such as an initial endoscopic exam when no symptoms are present or where the risk of malignancy seems likely to be limited to the rectal area, the rigid scope will suffice. In fact, even with the newer, high-tech flexible scopes now available, the rigid scope is still considered the best instrument for examining the lower 5 inches of the bowel, so much so that a number of doctors will use it to accompany examination with a flexible instrument.

When you discuss or schedule a sigmoidoscopic exam with your doctor, it's not unwise to ask about the kind of scope or scopes that will be used. If the physician intends to employ the rigid scope, you may want to inquire further about whether this is really the wisest kind of endoscopic exam for your situation, or whether your physician is merely unequipped to use the newer equipment. If that's the case, you're perfectly justified to ask the doctor to recommend a colleague who is able to perform the procedure using the more tolerable, and more complete, instruments.

Flexible Sigmoidoscopy

Recent advances in fiberoptic technology have led to the development of sigmoidoscopes that can explore much farther, and cause much less discomfort, than their predecessors. These instruments came into widespread use in the 1980s, and although many doctors are still not trained in the procedure or do not have the equipment, flexible sigmoidoscopies are available, at about the same cost as rigid sigmoidoscopies, in most parts of the country.

Sigmoidoscopies done with flexible scopes involve pretty much the same preparation and procedure as those performed with rigid scopes. The exam still is likely to take place in the doctor's office, but the bowel preparation may be a bit more extensive (because the flexible scope will probe farther, a larger portion of the colon will need to be clear). And because more of the colon will be examined, the procedure usually takes a little longer.

What makes this exam so much more tolerable is that the flexibility of the instrument means there is a relative lack of discomfort or outright pain. The scope is a long, pliant, lighted tube about the thickness of a finger, with a handle at the doctor's end. The tube contains a bendable fiberoptic system that allows the physician, using the handle, to guide or bend the far end of the instrument in any direction, leading the scope around the curves and bends of the colon and through the entire lower portion of the bowel. Bundles of fibers within the scope transmit a magnified image back to the doctor. The image is very clear, allowing the examiner to spot growths as small as an eighth of an inch. The instrument can also detect bowel inflammation caused by ulcerative colitis and sometimes can spot dysplasia, a suspicious buildup of cells along the bowel lining that may be an early indication of possible malignant activity. Frequently, the examiner will hook the scope up to a video monitor for the transmission of all these images, which readily allows photographing for later study.

Flexible sigmoidoscopes come in two lengths. The shorter is 10 to 14 inches and is easier for the physician to learn to use and more comfortable for the patient. The longer scope is 24 to 26 inches and can, obviously, explore farther into the colon to detect adenomatous growths, frequently as far as the transverse colon and even occasionally the cecum. About two-thirds of all cancers and polyps growing in the large bowel (or nearly three times the number detectable during rigid sigmoidoscopy) can be spotted using the longer scope, but a good 84 percent of those growths can also be found with the shorter tube. There is a slight possibility, as there is with the rigid scope, of false negative results; some polyps on the intestinal wall may be obscured if the bowel is not clear of mucus or fecal matter. But with the flexible scope, water, as well as air, can be sent through a separate channel in the tube to wash the bowel (or the scope's lens).

The flexible scope is also frequently equipped with accessories like scissors and forceps that are used to collect a tissue sample for biopsy, or even to remove polyps entirely. Generally, however, polyps are removed during colonoscopy rather than during sigmoidoscopy. In any event, if a polyp is detected, there's a 30 to 50 percent chance that at least one other polyp is growing elsewhere in the colon. So the discovery of any polyp requires follow-up with a full colonoscopic exam.

Because sigmoidoscopies are such a crucial part of colorectal cancer screening, concerns about the discomfort of the procedure should certainly not deter you from having the exam performed when necessary. Furthermore, the widespread use of flexible scopes ensures the availability of sigmoidoscopic tests that are remarkably discomfort free, all things considered. Plus, given the negligible time commitment required and the comparably low cost (particularly in comparison to the cost of cancer treatment), which medical insurance carriers have been increasingly willing to cover, there's no reason not to follow diligently the guidelines for a proper colorectal cancer screening program.

The American Cancer Society's general recommendation is that you receive two successive annual sigmoidoscopic exams once you turn fifty. If both these tests turn up no problem, you only need to follow up with exams every three to five years. Many doctors, however, assert that this recommendation might be overemphasizing cost effectiveness and suggest more frequent examinations—perhaps every other year—for patients willing to bear the extra expense, especially when they have a family history of colorectal cancer or are in another high-risk group. You can decide with your physician what your optimal program should be.

Colonoscopy

A full colonoscopic exam, which can explore the whole large bowel, is performed when the symptoms you experience or the results of prior screenings warrant inspection of the entire colon. In particular, colonoscopies are conducted if polyps have been found or are strongly suspected. These polyps, as we've seen, indicate a greater likelihood that others may be growing elsewhere in the bowel, in areas viewable only with a colonoscope. The vast majority of these growths can be removed altogether during this procedure without any need for abdominal surgery.

A colonoscope is similar in many ways to a flexible sigmoidoscope. It is quite a bit longer, however—usually about 5 feet—with a design and flexibility that allows the examiner to see the entire length of the large bowel. Like flexible sigmoidoscopes, the narrow colonoscope contains a fiberoptic viewing device and channels where air and water can be passed through to enlarge and clear the bowel, allowing easier passage of the instrument and better viewing. Through that same opening, tools are attached—forceps and a wire snare—used both to collect tissue samples for laboratory analysis and to remove adenomatous growths from the intestinal wall. At the examiner's end are knobs to maneuver the scope; a handle to open and close the forceps; and buttons to work the wire snare, pump air and water, and create suction for clearing away any obstructing material like blood, mucus, and feces.

A colonoscopic exam requires extensive preparation to clear the whole colon. You're usually instructed to follow a clear liquid diet for one to two days prior to the test and to take a strong laxative the evening before and one or more enemas in the final 3 to 4 hours. The exam itself is often performed at a hospital as an outpatient procedure; some doctors, however, will have you admitted to the hospital overnight and others may simply conduct the test in their office.

You will usually be given a sedative or tranquilizer that will keep you from feeling much discomfort while the procedure is taking place. Still, you remain at least semiconscious and may feel pressure in the stomach and abdomen as the scope is maneuvered around the bowel as well as the same feeling of fullness and urge to defecate and pass gas that is experienced during sigmoidoscopy. Because of the extensiveness of the procedure, it takes somewhat longer, anywhere from as little as 5 minutes in very experienced hands to more than 30 minutes if the doctor needs to collect tissue samples or remove a polyp. After the test is completed, you may be asked to remain a few hours for observation while the medication wears off.

During the exam, as the scope is advanced and withdrawn, the physician closely inspects the lining of the large intestine for growths or other suspicious activity. If a small polyp, which is very unlikely to be malignant, is spotted, it is usually removed. Using the knobs, buttons, and handles at the end of the instrument, the physician will extend a specially designed grasping forceps or wire basket from the colonoscopic tube and snip off a tumor projecting by a stalk from the surface of the bowel wall. Or the doctor can extend a wire snare in a loop from the tube, maneuver the loop around the polyp, and pass an electrical current through the wire to cauterize it, freeing the growth from the intestinal wall. Using suction to hold the detached polyp to the end of the instrument, the physician then withdraws the growth from the intestine and has it analyzed in the laboratory.

The colonoscope is also used to collect a small amount of tissue (with biopsy forceps) from growths too large to be removed during the exam. That tissue is then sent to a laboratory to be studied. Tumors of this size are much more likely to be cancerous and, in any event, will need to be surgically removed.

A colonoscopic exam is a particularly technical medical procedure that requires the expertise of a specialist, usually a gastroenterologist. (Colorectal and general surgeons also perform colonoscopies.) This physician must have thorough knowledge, extensive training, great skill in spotting very small polyps and cancers, and meticulous technique to avoid complications. The costs (customarily ranging from $500 to $700 or more, if a hospital stay is required, but medical insurance very often covers it), time, and slight risks involved make this a test reserved mostly for those people who have a particularly high likelihood of some kind of tumor growth—benign or malignant—in the colon. The possible complications include perforation of the bowel wall and some intestinal bleeding, but that happens very infrequently and the risks have been even further reduced with technological advances in the design of the colonoscope.

It must also be said that a colonoscopic exam is not completely foolproof. Some polyps may not be seen because of blind corners and mucosal forms and the scope may not be able to reach all the way to the cecum, at the far end of the colon. Furthermore, even with the use of air, water, and suction, improper preparation of the bowel, from not following the dietary restrictions, can adversely affect the results of the exam, as can the presence of blood in the intestine. And the passage of the colonoscope may be hindered in patients with inflammatory bowel disease, or who have had surgery or radiation treatment in the large intestine.

 Nevertheless, the colonoscopic exam remains a remarkably effective screening method for colorectal cancer, one able to detect 90 percent or more of all malignancies of the large bowel—and detect and remove the vast majority of polyps that could someday develop into cancer.

Barium Enema

Sometimes called a lower GI (for gastrointestinal) series, a barium enema is an X-ray study of the colon and rectum in which you are given an enema with barium sulfate, a contrast medium that provides clear fluoroscopic views of the bowel and reveals polyps and malignant tumors virtually anywhere in the large intestine. This exam is often given in conjunction with a colonoscopy or sigmoidoscopy to obtain an even more complete screening for colorectal cancer.

As with the endoscopic exams, a barium enema requires careful preparation to clear the bowel for the best possible X-ray images. Your doctor's office will give you the necessary materials or instruct you to purchase a preparation kit widely available at pharmacies. A liquid diet may be recommended. And, in addition to the laxatives or other special formulas, you'll probably also be told to take phosphosoda or tap-water enemas the evening before and morning of the test, repeating until the enema fluid expelled is clear.

The barium enema exam is usually performed by a radiologist, or X-ray technician, in a special laboratory. Before beginning, you may be given one final enema to make sure your bowel is completely clear. You'll start by lying down on your side as you are secured onto a tilting table. A catheter is inserted into the rectum through which the barium sulfate will be administered. As the barium is carefully passed into the bowel, the table will be rotated—you along with it—so the solution can completely coat the large intestine. The fluoroscope allows the examiner to see moving, rather than merely still, images of the bowel and to make sure the barium solution is covering the entire length. You may be assisted into various positions to help the passage of the barium through the colon.

The examiner will begin taking a series of X-ray pictures. It's important that you remain absolutely still as the X-ray film is exposed to ensure clearly focused images; you'll be told when you can move again. During the procedure, you may feel some cramping, and you will almost certainly feel a very strong urge to defecate. Controlling yourself while staying motionless is the big trick to the barium enema, but the examiner undoubtedly will be proceeding as briskly as possible.

Finally, you'll be given a bedpan—or helped to the bathroom—and be told to expel as much of the barium as possible (it won't be difficult). A thin film of barium will remain on the mucus lining of the intestine, so it's back on the table for another round of X rays.

This is what's known as a single-contrast barium enema. Frequently, it will be followed by a double-contrast, or air-contrast, study, developed in recent years to improve the accuracy of the exam and now considered by most physicians to be an integral part of the procedure. For that procedure, air is carefully introduced into the bowel through a catheter and one more set of X-ray images is taken. The air provides further contrast in the pictures, delineating more clearly possible growths in the bowel. During this part of the procedure in particular you are liable to experience moderate cramping.

The whole exam takes about 30 to 45 minutes. It is sometimes followed with another laxative or enema to clear out any barium solution from the bowel, because it may cause constipation. For the next couple of days, your stool will be white or light colored. The test also can cause dehydration, so be sure to drink plenty of fluids afterward. The test results, which are quickly available, may be impaired if the bowel is inadequately prepared (which will affect the quality of the photographed image) or if you have such trouble retaining the barium that the study must be abbreviated.

Barium enemas are more widely available and less expensive than colonoscopic exams—about $200, although in some areas the cost may be higher. The test is often given when a patient is unable—or unwilling—to undergo colonoscopy (although a colonoscopic exam accompanied by a sedative is usually more tolerable than a barium enema). The standard single-contrast study has been found to catch about two-thirds of early cancers; the double-contrast exam may be nearly as accurate as a colonoscopy, although there's some disagreement about that. A well-performed double-contrast barium enema will show virtually all growths larger than a fifth of an inch as well as many of those as small as an eighth of an inch, while a colonoscopic exam is still less likely to miss a lesion, routinely detecting even smaller growths. One advantage of the barium enema is that it virtually always allows examination of the cecum, unreachable in up to 10 percent of colonoscopic exams, although lesions there may occasionally be overlooked because the area is very difficult to inspect well. And barium enemas reveal polyps growing in areas of the bowel, particularly where the colon curves and flexes, that are difficult to inspect through endoscopy. In the final analysis, a barium enema is considered most useful when it's complemented by endoscopic screening. If a colonoscopic exam is not available in your area, you should still not hesitate to undergo a sigmoidoscopy in addition to the barium enema. Oftentimes, you will be scheduled to take both exams the same day, which, while not making for a particularly enjoyable morning, gets it all over with at once and, more important, provides your doctor with as complete a picture as possible of exactly what may be going on in your large bowel.

All these diagnostic exams and procedures, as we've said, are most informative and reliable when they are performed in conjunction with one another. With this kind of complementary scrutiny, you are very likely to discover if you have colorectal cancer even at an early and highly curable stage. One mathematical model determined that if these exams were performed together on a regular basis, mortality from cancer of the large bowel could be decreased by more than 90 percent. And it's almost as likely that you'll learn about any precancerous activity that merits further attention and observation, which may prevent you from developing cancer altogether.

Your Screening Program

The particular combination of tests best suited to you or to a member of your family, like the degree to which you are at risk of colorectal cancer, depends on several factors, including your age, health background, family history, and the symptoms (if any) you may have experienced. Those in a high-risk group, in particular, require an individualized regimen. By consulting with your doctor and with other specialists, you should be able to determine a screening program that is neither too lax nor excessively fastidious, one that will provide you with maximum protection.

Remember that because results of these procedures can be inaccurate or misleading, it's important to be examined further if you continue to experience any symptoms. Don't wait until your next checkup to have these symptoms evaluated. Putting off a visit or phone call to the doctor can jeopardize your chances of being cured.

Furthermore, even when accurate, negative results from any of these tests do not guarantee that you won't develop cancer, or precancerous polyps, in the future. So it's every bit as important to continue to be screened regularly.

These are standard general guidelines for screening regimens. Again, your doctor may recommend some variation on these programs based on the particulars of your health and family background, and your physician's own position on the usefulness and accuracy of the various exams.

SCREENING REGIMENS

- If you are not in a high-risk group:
    Annual digital rectal exam, once you turn forty.
    Annual fecal occult blood test, once you turn fifty.
    Sigmoidoscopy every three to five years after two successive negative exams conducted one year apart, once you turn fifty (some physicians recommend more frequent screening—sigmoidoscopy every other year, beginning by age forty).
- If you have a family history of colorectal cancer (one or more close relatives who have had the disease):
    Screening should begin by age thirty-five, or earlier if there is a particularly high incidence of colorectal cancer in your family.
    Annual <u>fecal occult blood test</u>.
    Annual <u>digital rectal exam</u>.
    <u>Flexible sigmoidoscopy</u> every three to five years, if previous exams have been negative (more often if there is a

particularly high incidence of colorectal cancer in your family).

- If your family has a history of a genetic cancer syndrome (Lynch syndrome I or II):

  Screening should begin by age thirty-five or earlier (some physicians recommend beginning regular screening as early as the teen years).

  Annual fecal occult blood test.

  Frequent—even annual—colonoscopy or sigmoidoscopy.

  Air-contrast barium enema every three to five years.

- If your family has a history of familial polyposis syndrome:

  Fecal occult blood test three times annually starting at age ten.

  Sigmoidoscopy two times annually starting at age fifteen (the test is difficult for young children), provided no symptoms develop earlier.

  Colonoscopy and barium enema at age twenty (as a baseline to measure changes against); annually thereafter.

  If familial polyposis has been diagnosed, and the colon, but not the rectum, has been removed, sigmoidoscopy is necessary every six months.

- If you have had ulcerative colitis for more than ten years:

  Flexible sigmoidoscopy or colonoscopy every one to two years—more often if the condition is severe—with tissue biopsies for detecting dysplasia.

- If you have a history of polyps or previous colorectal cancer:

  Sigmoidoscopy or colonoscopy every one to three years.

  Air-contrast barium enema in addition is also recommended.

- *For women,* if you have a history of cancer of the breast or reproductive organs:

  Screening should begin in your thirties.

  Annual fecal occult blood test.

  Annual digital rectal exam.

  Sigmoidoscopy every three to five years.

A Case Study: Ronald Reagan

To illustrate the details of screening procedures—what they might reveal and what they might miss—and the choices doctors make in specific circumstances about which exams to administer and when, let's look at the real-life experience of perhaps the most famous colorectal cancer patient, former President Ronald Reagan.

Reagan's background suggested he was at least at moderately high risk for colorectal cancer. When he learned of benign and malignant tumor activity in his large bowel, Reagan was in his early seventies, the age at which colorectal cancer is most prevalent. Unknown to him at the time, he also had a family background of this type of cancer; his brother had surgery to remove a cancerous tumor from the same part of the colon that Reagan's malignancy was located, the same month as Reagan's operation. Plus, he experienced signs and symptoms that warranted thorough screening for the possible presence of a malignancy in the large bowel.

REAGAN'S HEALTH PROFILE

Age at Diagnosis:	Seventy-four.
Weight:	Near ideal weight.
General Health:	Good (prior incidence of hyperplastic polyps; recovery essentially complete from 1981 gunshot wound).
Diet:	Typical senior statesmen's diet (frequent heavy banquet fare, occasional missed meals; is also known for liking his steak).
Exercise:	Sporadic (he had the White House gym, but probably wasn't using it daily; got lots of outdoor exercise during visits to his California ranch).

Family Background of Colorectal Cancer:	Younger brother had surgery for cancerous tumor in the colon around the time Reagan's cancer was diagnosed; Reagan and his doctors had not known of his brother's disease.

At age seventy-three, Ronald Reagan was having his regular physical exam in May 1984, when his doctors, while performing a sigmoidoscopy using a flexible scope, detected a small hyperplastic polyp growing about 16 inches into his colon. Removing the growth with the instrument and finding it to be benign, they did not perform any further follow-up tests at that time, neither an air-contrast barium enema nor a full colonoscopic exam.

Ten months later, in March 1985, Reagan had another routine general checkup. As part of it, his doctors obtained four stool samples to test for the presence of occult blood. Two of these tests turned out to be positive and two negative. The president's physicians thought the positive tests might be false. They advised Reagan to take the test again, making sure to avoid red meat and certain other foods for several days beforehand. All six of this second round of stool samples were negative.

Nevertheless, another sigmoidoscopic exam performed that March revealed a second tiny polyp, about a seventh of an inch in diameter and located 18 inches into the colon. At that size, the growth was undoubtedly benign; the doctors saw little need to remove it right away. This time, however, the physicians wanted to examine the president's entire colon for the possible presence of other tumors growing beyond the range of the sigmoidoscope or any polyps that may have been missed in the previous tests. The polyp already detected would be removed during the exam.

Four months later, on July 12, 1985, the president checked into the hospital to undergo that colonoscopy. Then, doctors were able to detect yet another polyp, this one a large villous adenoma, about 2 inches in diameter, growing in the president's cecum. This growth was too large to be removed with the colonoscope. And the size and type of polyp strongly indicated the tumor was likely to be malignant. Surgery would be needed.

But not necessarily right away. The tumor wasn't obstructing or perforating the bowel, so this wasn't an emergency situation. The operation could be safely delayed a short period until a more convenient time in the president's schedule opened up. Reagan chose to go right ahead with the surgery. He remained in the hospital that night, and X rays and CAT scans were performed on his liver and lungs to look for any potential spread of malignancy. None was found. The next morning, Reagan underwent abdominal surgery and had the tumor and a surrounding segment of the intestine removed. The news was announced to the world. The president remained in the hospital for the next several days. A biopsy of the excised polyp, meanwhile, determined that it was indeed cancerous. The indications were, nevertheless, that the surgery was entirely successful and that there had been no spread of the cancer to other parts of the body. Reagan returned home, and his bowel habits returned to normal.

To sum up: It was cancer, but the operation appeared to be entirely successful and was performed, apparently, before the cancer had spread elsewhere.

This was still a very serious illness. The cancer had developed past the earliest stages, when it is almost always curable, to a point at which the chances of recurrence become greater. However, Reagan, it's reported, handled the news of his diagnosis with excellent spirits and great optimism, factors that are elemental to successful recovery.

The country, on the other hand, panicked somewhat. In a predictable, but entirely erroneous, response to the word *cancer,* many people were even ready to write Reagan off. Statistics vastly inflating the president's odds against survival were regularly bandied about. And many expressed doubts—despite the fact that the vast majority of cancer patients are able entirely to resume their normal lives after surgery—that he would be able to continue at his job.

However, it has now been more than five years since Reagan's cancer surgery. He is alive and there has been no word of recurrence of the disease. Reagan seems to be enjoying his retirement free of cancer.

The former president's experience demonstrates the benefits—and also the drawbacks—of the various exams used to detect colorectal cancer and its precursors. If they didn't prevent him from developing a malignancy, these procedures ultimately served him well; his disease was discovered at a point at which it could still be cured. Although earlier tests missed Reagan's cancer, follow-up examinations caught it in time for surgical treatment to have, apparently, been entirely successful.

That's not to say the exams wound up being foolproof. The results of eight of ten of Reagan's fecal blood tests were negative, even though at that very time he had a large cancerous tumor growing in the bowel. And the two sigmoidoscopic exams he received could not reach far enough into the bowel to detect the malignant tumor.

There's also the margin of human error to consider as well. Even well-trained examiners can miss, or misinterpret, warning signs during these tests. They can also make perfectly reasonable choices for a screening procedure that will still wind up not being thorough enough, overlooking malignancies in the colon and rectum. That's why it's so important not to be complacent if test results reveal nothing. It doesn't mean you should doubt any good news, but you should not let that good news diminish your diligence and ignore persistent warning signs and the need to keep going in for exams in the future.

President Reagan's doctors seemed willing to accept the results of tests that showed no sign of cancer, even though it turns out a malignancy was actually present. And they opted against performing other exams that might well have spotted the cancer sooner. These were not unreasonable or imprudent decisions; it is just that, in hindsight, they probably turned out to have been the wrong ones. Nevertheless, once the cancer was discovered, many medical experts publicly criticized Reagan's doctors. They argued that the president's physicians should have performed a full colonoscopy, or at least a barium enema, when the first polyp was discovered in 1984 and wondered why he wasn't given those exams as soon as the second polyp was found the following year.

Well, the size of the tumor in Reagan's cecum indicated it had been growing for several years, and so would have likely been spotted earlier if he had undergone an exam of the entire bowel. But it's impossible to say if more aggressive screening would have actually caught the polyp before it became malignant, thus preventing Reagan's cancer altogether.

As you go on to make decisions about your own—and your family's—health care, remember the experience of Ronald Reagan. Remember that anyone can develop colorectal cancer, so it's vital not to overlook the warning signs, even in a young person at very low risk. Cancer, yes, is unlikely, but the diagnosis of the actual problem may provide ample reason to follow cancer prevention practices now and quite possibly avoid cancer in the future. And remember that even a president of the United States, with some of the best doctors in attendance and the most closely observed body in the world, can have his cancer entirely overlooked during examinations. But if one perseveres with a sensible screening program, even cancer missed earlier on can still be detected and successfully treated.

7

Treatment and Outlook for the Future

"I didn't have cancer," Ronald Reagan said in one of his first interviews after receiving surgery to remove a malignant tumor, "I had something inside of me that had cancer in it, and it was removed."

Reagan displayed an optimistic mind-set that too few of us have when it comes to cancer, a kind of hopeful attitude instrumental in successful cancer recovery. Yes, it's important not to let blind optimism dissuade you from caution, from acknowledging the possibility of a not-so-favorable outcome. But Reagan wasn't being unrealistic; he has, according to all accounts, observed a prudent follow-up regimen for former colorectal cancer patients, remaining on his guard for a possible recurrence of the disease. But he did not allow the foreboding weight of the word *cancer* to unnerve him. It's a serious condition, but it doesn't define my whole being, Reagan was saying; my doctors seemed to have treated it successfully, and we will be watching closely from now on for any signs of it coming back again.

So many people are so afraid of this disease that they delay seeking treatment. And that's the worst thing you can do. Colorectal cancer detected in its earliest stages is curable more than 90 percent of the time, and delaying medical care only jeopardizes your chances.

Others are as afraid of the cure as they are of the disease. Too many people mistakenly believe that the removal of any cancerous growth in the bowel leaves you an invalid: no longer in control of your bowel functions; a slave to a humiliating, lifelong colostomy regimen; unable to work, enjoy sex, or play sports; and uncomfortable in public. Nothing is further from the truth.

Let's look at the facts and dispel the untrue rumors. What if you *do* have colorectal cancer?

Assessment and Prognosis

The outlook for an individual with colorectal cancer depends on several factors: age and general health, the location of the tumor, certain features of the cancer cell, and especially, the extent of the malignancy's spread.

Once a tumor has been discovered in the colon or rectum, several tests will be performed:

- A biopsy of tumor tissues, to determine if it is cancerous in the first place.
- Further blood tests.
- X rays of parts of the body to which the cancer may have spread.
- CAT scans or nuclear magnetic resonance (NMR) imaging (three-dimensional X rays) of the abdominal area.

These tests will determine the stage of the disease. The assessment, or "staging," of colorectal cancer is based on a system first devised by British pathologist Cuthbert Dukes in 1932, and since somewhat modified. (The disease may also be rated by the less-widely used TNM classification system, recently developed by the American Joint Committee on Cancer.) Table 5 is a brief overview of the Dukes classification.

Table 5. Dukes Classification of Colorectal Cancer Stages

Category	Definition	Current Five-Year Survival Rates (percent)
Stage A	Cancer is very superficial, only slightly penetrating bowel wall; little risk that cancer has spread to other sites; almost never fatal when detected at this stage.	90
Stage B	Tumor has begun to penetrate into muscle layer, but not into lymph nodes.	60–75
Stage C	Tumor has penetrated through the intestine, into regional lymph nodes; cure is more likely if fewer than three nodes are involved; cancer will recur in about 55 percent of cases.	30–40
Stage D	Cancer has spread to liver or other organs.	5

The low survival rates for the more advanced stages of colorectal cancer may give you reason to pause. The prognosis in those cases is, frankly, not usually encouraging (although, remember that even then, a fatal outcome is not inevitable). But as we've seen, cancer can almost always be detected in its earliest stages if you take the proper precautions. *What these statistics should do is help you see even more clearly the wisdom of regular screening and of reporting any symptoms.* Currently about 40 percent of colorectal cancers are detected in the early stages, when the prognosis for cure and survival is very good. But that figure could be *substantially* higher—one study even suggests more than 90 percent—if more people underwent the recommended screening programs.

Physicians do not have to wait for complete staging of the disease before treatment can begin. A polyp removed during colonoscopy or surgery is often determined only later to be malignant.

The physician can predict the likelihood of a tumor being cancerous, as we've seen, based on its type and size—and can treat it accordingly. When a polyp is too large to be able to be removed with a colonoscope, that treatment usually does mean surgery.

Surgery

Although surgery can be a frightening experience, the surgery performed to treat cancer of the large bowel is invariably much less drastic—and much less risky—than most people imagine. In the first place, it's usually far less extensive than you might think. It's rarely necessary for the entire colon and rectum to be removed. And a permanent colostomy, the most feared aftereffect of abdominal surgery, is currently required less than 15 percent of the time.

Abdominal surgery for colorectal cancer is rarely an emergency procedure. Although the discovery of any polyp is a serious matter, unless the intestine is obstructed or the growth has perforated the bowel, there is little harm in waiting even as long as several weeks. The detection of a polyp during sigmoidoscopy warrants a full colonoscopic follow-up anyway to locate any other possible tumors growing farther up the colon. So the physician will frequently suggest waiting until the entire colon is examined, using, as we've discussed, the scope itself to remove the smaller growths.

To remove tumors too large to be handled with the colonoscope, the surgeon and patient may choose to go right ahead with surgery, because the bowel is already adequately prepared for the procedure. Or further tests may be performed prior to the surgery to determine the possible spread of any malignancy and whether preoperative radiotherapy might be useful and to ascertain whether an older patient is in good enough health to undergo the operation at that time.

Surgery for colorectal cancer involves the *resection* of the diseased portion of the large intestine. The surgeon, in what's sometimes referred to as the "no-touch procedure," will usually remove the section of the bowel containing the tumor, plus a wide margin of healthy tissue around it. As a typical example, in Reagan's cancer operation, doctors removed about an 18-inch section of the large intestine, the cecum, and a portion of the ascending colon.

This operation is called a segmental resection. The excised portion of the bowel itself is not opened, reducing the possibility of infection and keeping the tumor itself intact so that no cancerous cells will be shed and remain in the abdominal area. The surgeon will also generally remove some of the surrounding lymph nodes, the major route of cancer spread, that drain the area, to have them examined for signs of advanced disease.

For more widespread or advanced cancers, there often are still other surgical techniques that save a portion of the colon as well. These include a *hemicolectomy,* in which either the entire right side or the entire left side of the colon is removed, and a *subtotal colectomy,* resection of the entire colon except for the rectum.

For rectal tumors, if there's no indication of cancer spread, the surgeon may remove only the growth itself, or perhaps a small wedge of the rectum encompassing the tumor and some surrounding tissue.

In most cases, the healthy, albeit severed, ends of the intestine are then reconnected right during the operation, a procedure known as *anastomosis.* The abdominal wall is then closed, and the surgery is complete. The intestine, even though it is now shorter, will function normally. And the patient will have no lingering change in bowel functions at all.

In some cases, however, when the patient has an increased

risk of bowel infection, inflammation, obstruction, or other problems, the intestine may need a chance to heal, and the surgeon will not perform anastomosis at the time of cancer surgery. Instead, he or she will perform a temporary colostomy, creating an artificial opening in the abdominal wall, called a *stoma,* through which a portion of the colon is attached for the elimination of waste. (The waste is collected in a plastic bag worn outside the body.) Once the patient has had the chance to heal, the surgeon will reconnect the intestine, restoring normal bowel function. It's only when the ends of the intestine can never be reconnected—when, for example, the entire rectum is removed or the surgeon was unable to preserve the sphincter muscle— that a permanent colostomy is necessary.

Many people automatically associate colorectal cancer with colostomies. The reality, however, is that they are now the exception rather than the rule. Once a common consequence of cancer of the rectum or descending colon, at present, fewer than one in seven colorectal patients require permanent colostomy (or ileostomy, when the lower part of the small intestine is used to form the stoma because the entire colon and rectum have been removed).

Several developments over the last twenty years have made this possible:

- Surgical techniques have improved, allowing for easier reconnection of the intestine.
- Alternatives to removal of the entire rectum in treating rectal cancer are increasingly available; one new procedure being studied involves electrocoagulation, the use of electric currents to destroy tumors in the rectum.
- Colorectal cancers are appearing more often in higher parts of the colon than before, where reconnection of the bowel is almost always feasible.

This isn't to guarantee that any colorectal cancer patient these days will avoid a permanent colostomy. Nor is it to say that living with one is the tragedy that many people envision. A colostomy is a lifesaving measure that allows an individual to continue leading an otherwise perfectly normal—and healthy—existence. It is not as disruptive as you'd think, and you can carry on in work, sports, sex, and all the other features of everyday life pretty much the way you had before.

The recovery process from colorectal cancer surgery is relatively easy and routine. The patient will usually remain in the hospital for about eight days (longer if a colostomy has been performed), during which time he or she will start eating solid foods again, normal bowel functions will return, and any post-surgery discomfort will abate. The hospital stay is followed by further convalescence at home; in general, a patient can return to work within six weeks, and even resume part-time work while still in the hospital.

It's also during the recovery period that the physician will discuss with the patient the disease prognosis. Right after performing the operation, the doctor will be able to describe the visible extent of the tumor. Later, when the biopsy results are obtained, he or she will know for certain whether the tumor was malignant. The other blood tests and X rays along with examination of the excised lymph nodes will have helped further to determine whether the disease has spread. At that point the extent of the condition can be pretty precisely concluded. And the physician and patient can then decide if any further treatment might be warranted.

Chemotherapy

Drug treatment, called adjuvant or supplemental chemotherapy, is occasionally recommended for colorectal cancer patients following surgery. The chemotherapy is sometimes effective at killing undetectable cancer cells that remain in the body after the operation. Usually performed on people with more advanced disease, drug treatment may also be used to provide added protection even if there is no evidence that cancer has spread beyond the bowel.

Although it has hardly been a panacea, adjuvant chemotherapy has frequently improved both disease-free survival and overall survival time among cancer patients whose prognosis is poor. The drugs are administered using a variety of methods: orally, intravenously, or both. New techniques of infusion as well as potentially more effective drug combinations are being investigated. People undergoing chemotherapy treatment for colorectal cancer receive the drugs regularly, the dose, drug combination, and schedule varying from patient to patient, over a period of time as long as several years.

Radiotherapy

It is sometimes beneficial for colorectal patients to undergo radiotherapy (X-ray treatment) prior to abdominal surgery, to attempt to shrink the tumor and improve the chances for the operation to be successful. Radiation therapy may also be performed after surgery, in an effort to block the growth of malignant cells that remain in the area after the operation, and thus reduce the possibility of a recurrence of cancer.

Radiotherapy is more frequently used—and has thus far been more effective—for treatment of cancers of the rectum, where recurrence is far more likely. In some cases, but only rarely so far, it may even be performed in the place of surgery. One process now being tried is called endocavitary irradiation. Here a special proctoscope is fitted with an X-ray tube. The physician then can see inside the rectum while performing the procedure and aim the rays directly at the tumor. This method, along with several others being investigated, may hold future promise for treatment of malignancies growing even higher in the bowel as well.

Recurrence

Colorectal cancer may recur at, or near, the site of the original tumor. An entirely new malignancy may develop elsewhere in the colon or rectum. And the disease may spread to other organs, especially the liver.

Anyone who has had colorectal cancer is, as we discussed in chapter 2, at increased risk—approximately a 5 to 10 percent chance—of developing the disease again. People whose cancer is detected at an early stage are more unlikely to have a recurrence of the original malignancy or to develop cancer elsewhere in the body. The chances are, however, greater if the disease is not detected until a more advanced stage. Nevertheless, it's vital that *all* people who have had cancer of the large bowel be followed carefully and screened regularly, so a recurrence or the development of a new malignancy can be detected as soon as possible.

Along with the other examinations already described in detail, many people who have had colorectal cancer are regularly given a CEA test. This is a simple blood test that measures the concentration of a substance called carcinoembryonic antigen (CEA). A rise in the level of the antigen in the blood may indicate the presence of a new cancerous tumor, often before there are any other signs of the disease. The CEA test is not always reliable; the antigen level may remain normal even when a malignancy has developed, or it may rise for some other reason. Because of this, this test is not currently used to screen individuals who have never had the disease. But several studies have demonstrated its value as an early indicator of tumor recurrence.

What the Future Holds

We discussed in chapter 3 what the great strides being made in genetic research may mean for the prevention of colorectal cancer. With these advances, we are already, as we've seen, beginning to detect more effectively those people who are at an increased risk of developing the disease—who can then proceed to follow a program of healthy eating, regular outdoor exercise, and regular screening as well as to watch closely for any warning signs. And we've seen how scientists in the not-too-distant future may even be able to repair damaged genes that cause malignant activity in the cell.

There are also enormous strides being made in the treatment of colorectal cancer. For those patients whose cancer was detected in an early stage, abdominal surgery, once again, is remarkably effective, resulting in a complete cure the vast majority of the time. And continuing advancements and refinements in surgical techniques and preoperative and postoperative care are making this form of treatment still more effective.

The outlook for patients with more advanced stages of the disease is getting brighter as well, with innovative developments in chemotherapy, radiotherapy, and immunotherapy showing great potential. The survival rates continue to improve, and that's largely because patients in clinical trials are obtaining the benefits of these new, ever-improving methods of treating colorectal cancer.

Chemotherapy

Scientists are busily looking for ways to improve the effectiveness of chemotherapeutic techniques used in treating colorectal cancer. Many studies currently under way are determining the most effective dosages and treatment schedules and even new and more powerful ways to administer the drugs. One innovative method now being investigated is the use of a catheter to infuse the chemotherapeutic agents, exposing affected areas directly to a high concentration of anticancer drugs without requiring them to circulate throughout the body.

At the same time, researchers are also developing and testing the merits of new anticancer agents and drug combinations. And there are several encouraging ones already coming into use.

One drug combination that is receiving a lot of attention is 5-fluorouracil (5-FU) and levamisole. 5-FU has been a standard chemotherapeutic agent used in the treatment of colorectal cancer for more than twenty-five years. But when administered with levamisole, a drug commonly used to rid farm animals of worms, it may be even more effective. In a study of 1,300 people with cancer that had spread to the lymph nodes, this combination was found to reduce the death rates by 33 percent and decrease the risk of recurrence by 41 percent. The patients began this therapy from three to five weeks following surgery, and the side effects experienced were not severe. Cancer specialists and the National Institutes of Health have now endorsed the use of 5-FU and levamisole together on patients who have had surgery for advanced colorectal cancer.

Another potential anticancer agent that shows early promise is a drug called 9-AC. This substance, derived from a Chinese tree, has been found to cause rapid and dramatic shrinking—and even complete disappearance—of human colon cancers that were transplanted into mice. As of this writing, the drug still awaits Food and Drug Administration approval for testing in humans. 9-AC is a variation of a drug that had been tested in clinical trials for its effect against colorectal cancer in the early 1970s but proved to be too toxic. But there has been no evidence thus far of any significant adverse effects from 9-AC in the animal studies, and the National Cancer Institute considers it a priority drug for further testing in animals, and if the indications continue to be positive, eventually it will be tested in people with advanced colorectal cancer.

Radiotherapy

A great deal of research is currently being done to help clarify the value of radiotherapy in the treatment of colorectal cancer. Several clinical trials, for example, are attempting to determine whether giving low doses of radiation before surgery to patients even with early-stage tumors can further improve the results. For people with more advanced cancer, much of the focus is on what's called the "sandwich technique," a combination of pre-operative and postoperative radiation treatment. New studies have indeed indicated that it does reduce the risk of local recurrence of the disease. Another relatively new treatment technique, called intraoperative radiation, is also currently being evaluated in clinical trials. With this treatment, radiation is given during surgery, when the tumor is exposed and the surrounding normal tissue can be shielded.

Some of the most encouraging findings are coming from clinical trials involving a combination of radiotherapy and chemotherapy. Patients in these programs are being shown to have reduced recurrence of the disease and better chances for survival than if they had been treated with surgery alone. What's more, as scientists continue to determine more effective combinations of anticancer agents to use in the chemotherapy portion, we will likely see even greater benefits from this kind of treatment program.

Immunotherapy

Also known as *biotherapy,* this realm of treatment attempts to use the body's immune system to delay or prevent the recurrence of colorectal cancer. Medical professionals have identified several natural substances and developed a number of synthetic ones called biologic-response modifiers. These substances can help restore, boost, or direct the body's normal defense mechanisms to fight cancer growth.

Colorectal cancer specialists, for example, have been looking closely at the potential of interleukin-2 (IL-2), a biologic-response modifier that stimulates the growth of *lymphocytes,* white blood cells produced by the immune system. Researchers are finding that IL-2, either injected into the bloodstream or infused directly into the lower abdomen, may hinder cancerous activity in the bowel. Other biologic-response modifiers that are currently being investigated include several different types of interferon, an antiviral protein able to draw immune cells that can destroy cancer.

And there is a whole class of biologic-response modifiers called *monoclonal antibodies,* substances that can locate tumor cells in the body and bind to them. Monoclonal antibodies are either used alone or, perhaps more effectively, used with various other cancer-killing materials to deliver drugs, toxins, or radioactivity directly to the cells.

The merits of all these, and other, substances are now being studied extensively in clinical trials. Some of the initial results have been encouraging, suggesting that within the next few years immunotherapy may be playing a critical role in the treatment of cancer of the large bowel.

Your Own Future: A Final Word

The advances made in finding better treatments, and even a cure, for colorectal cancer, encouraging as they are, can never be rapid enough. The good news is that for the vast majority of us—even those at high risk—the weapons we need to fight the disease are already at hand. *That is, as long as we know what they are and how to use them.* Whatever the future holds for colorectal cancer research, you can be the master of your own—and your family's—fate.

This book has told you how to begin. The place to start is determining if you are at risk . . . and recognizing you can still do something about it. Of course, no one, from what we currently know, is entirely risk free. But in learning how and when you face an increased likelihood of developing the disease, you can determine the importance of doing the things that will limit, and even reduce, this likelihood. That means adapting your eating habits and other lifestyle practices. It means being aware of the warning signs of the disease . . . and being willing to report them promptly. And it means being willing to undergo regular screening, the kind of exams that just might save your life.

There are, of course, two vital partners in this whole lifesaving enterprise: your family and your doctor.

We all have a responsibility for the lives and well-being of those closest to us. That's never so true as when we and our relatives face a common, dangerous threat like cancer. Yes, you can as a family be at risk of colorectal cancer. But just as certainly, and just as crucially, you can work together as a family to reduce that risk: to make nutritious, well-balanced meals together; to plan outdoor activities together; to discuss together other ways to live a healthier life; and to get together to encourage reluctant family members to see the doctor.

Doctors, to be sure, don't have all the answers, and that can be frustrating. "Will I get cancer?" "Will I be cured?" You want to know exactly what your chances are; doctors hesitate to predict, and for good reason.

This book has included a lot of statistics, many presented with no small degree of trepidation as to how they will be interpreted. The idea is not to become obsessed with determining your precise odds, with trying to figure out if you have a 13 percent chance of getting the disease or a 14 percent chance, as though colorectal cancer and its prevention were some kind of horse race to bet on. The idea, rather, is to acknowledge if you are affected by any of the health, genetic, or environmental factors. And then to go ahead and start doing the things that will count, the things that will indeed lower the odds.

The time to start is now.

8

Resources

The National Cancer Institute (NCI)

This federal agency, a division of the Department of Health and Human Services' National Institutes of Health, sponsors a nationwide toll-free telephone service:

> Cancer Information Service (CIS)
> (1)–(800) 4–CANCER (422–6237)
> In Alaska: (1)–(800) 638–6070
> In Hawaii: (1)–(800) 524–1234

Trained, nonphysician information specialists, including Spanish-speaking operators, are available to answer questions from cancer patients and their families, as well as from the general public.

You may also call the number to order NCI publications free of charge. Some of the materials of special interest to those concerned about colorectal cancer include:

Cancer Prevention Research: Chemotherapy and Diet

Cancer Rates and Risks

Chemotherapy and You: A Guide to Self-Help During Treatment

Diet, Nutrition and Cancer Prevention: Food Choices (includes recipes)

Eating Hints: Recipes and Tips for Better Nutrition During Cancer Treatment

Everything Doesn't Cause Cancer

Good News, Better News, Best News: Cancer Prevention

Research Report: Cancer of the Colon and Rectum

Services Available for People with Cancer: National and Regional Organizations

Taking Time: Support for People with Cancer

What Are Clinical Trials All About

What You Need to Know About Colon and Rectal Cancer

These and other publications may also be ordered by writing to the NCI:

Public Inquiries Section
Office of Cancer Communications

National Cancer Institute
Building 31, Room 10A16
9000 Rockville Pike
Bethesda, MD 20892

In addition, the NCI maintains a database of the latest published information about cancer. CIS operators will access this source for callers to perform a search on a particular subject or cancer site, and will send along the relevant materials on request.

Comprehensive Cancer Centers

The following health facilities have received official designation by the NCI as comprehensive cancer centers. Each of these facilities supports extensive cancer prevention and research programs, participates in coordinated national clinical trials, and maintains the ability to perform advanced diagnostic and treatment procedures.

Alabama
Comprehensive Cancer
   Center
University of Alabama in
   Birmingham
University Station
Birmingham, Alabama 35294
(205) 934–6612

California
UCLA Jonsson
Comprehensive Cancer
   Center, UCLA Center for
   Health Sciences
10833 Leconte Avenue
Los Angeles, California
   90024
(213) 206–6017 (public)

University of Southern
   California
Comprehensive Cancer
   Center
2025 Zonal Avenue
Los Angeles, California
   90033
(213) 224–6600

Connecticut
Yale University
  Comprehensive Cancer
  Center
333 Cedar Street
New Haven, Connecticut
  06510
(203) 436–3779

District of Columbia
Howard University Cancer
  Center
2041 Georgia Avenue NW
Washington, DC 20060
(202) 636–7697

Vincent T. Lombardi Cancer
  Research Center
Georgetown University
  Medical Center
3800 Reservoir Road NW
Washington, DC 20007
(202) 625–7066

Florida
Comprehensive Cancer
  Center for the State of
  Florida
University of Miami School
  of Medicine
P.O. Box 016960-D8-4
Miami, Florida 33103
(305) 547–7707 ext. 203

Illinois
Northwestern University
  Cancer Center

Health Sciences Building
303 East Chicago Avenue
Chicago, Illinois 60611
(312) 266–5250

Illinois Cancer Council
36 South Wabash Avenue
  Suite 700
Chicago, Illinois 60603
(312) 346–9813 or
  (1)–(800) 4–CANCER

Rush-Presbyterian-St. Luke's
  Medical Center
1753 West Congress Parkway
Chicago, Illinois 60612
(312) 942–6642

Cancer Research Center
University of Chicago
5841 South Maryland
  Avenue
Chicago, Illinois 60637
(312) 962–6180

University of Illinois
P.O. Box 6998
Chicago, Illinois 60608
(312) 996–8843 or
  996–6666

Maryland
The Johns Hopkins Oncology
  Center
600 North Wolfe Street
Baltimore, Maryland 21205
(301) 955–3636

Massachusetts
Dana-Farber Cancer Institute
44 Binney Street
Boston, Massachusetts 02115
(617) 732–3150 or
 732–3000

Michigan
Comprehensive Cancer
 Center of Metropolitan
 Detroit
110 East Warren Avenue
Detroit, Michigan 48201
(313) 833–0710 ext. 356 or
 393

Minnesota
Mayo Comprehensive Cancer
 Center
200 First Street SW
Rochester, Minnesota 55901
(507) 284–8285

New York
Roswell Park Memorial
 Institute
666 Elm Street
Buffalo, New York 14263
(716) 845–2300

Columbia University
 Comprehensive Cancer
 Center
College of Physicians &
 Surgeons

701 West 168 Street
New York, New York 10032
(212) 694–6900

Memorial Sloan-Kettering
 Cancer Center
1275 York Avenue
New York, New York 10021
(212) 794–7984

North Carolina
Duke Comprehensive Cancer
 Center
P.O. Box 3814
Duke University Medical
 Center
Durham, North Carolina
 27710
(919) 684–2282

Ohio
The Ohio State University
 Comprehensive Cancer
 Center
410 West 12th Avenue, Suite
 302
Columbus, Ohio 43210
(614) 422–5022

Pennsylvania
Fox Chase/University of
 Pennsylvania
 Comprehensive Cancer
 Center
7701 Burholme Avenue

Philadelphia, Pennsylvania
   19111
(215) 728–2717

Texas
The University of Texas
   Health System Cancer
   Center
M. D. Anderson Hospital
   and Tumor Institute
Box 90
6723 Bertner Avenue
Houston, Texas 77030
(713) 792–3030

Washington
Fred Hutchinson Cancer
   Research Center
1124 Columbia Street
Seattle, Washington 98104
(206) 292–6301

Wisconsin
The University of Wisconsin
   Clinical Cancer Center
600 Highland Avenue
Madison, Wisconsin 53706
(608) 263–8600

The American Cancer Society

This national voluntary organization furnishes information on all sites of cancer, offers a wide variety of services to patients and their families, and conducts extensive research and education programs. There are 57 regional divisions and nearly 3,000 local offices throughout the country.

National Headquarters
American Cancer Society
1599 Clifton Road NE
Atlanta, GA 30329
(1)–(800) 227–2345

Listed below are the chartered divisions of the American Cancer Society:

Alabama Division, Inc.
402 Office Park Drive
Suite 300
Birmingham, Alabama 35223
(205) 879–2242

Alaska Division, Inc.
406 West Fireweed Lane
Suite 204
Anchorage, Alaska 99503
(907) 277–8696

Arizona Division, Inc.
2929 East Thomas Road
Phoenix, Arizona 85016
(602) 224–0524

Arkansas Division, Inc.
901 North University
Little Rock, Arkansas 77202
(501) 664–3480

California Division, Inc.
1710 Webster Street
P.O. Box 2061
Oakland, California 94612
(415) 893–7900

Colorado Division, Inc.
2255 South Oneida
P.O. Box 24669

Denver, Colorado 80224
(303) 758–2030

Connecticut Division, Inc.
Barnes Park South
14 Village Lane
Wallingford, Connecticut
   06492
(203) 265–7161

Delaware Division, Inc.
92 Read's Way
New Castle, Delaware 19720
(302) 324–4227

District of Columbia
   Division, Inc.
1825 Connecticut Avenue,
   NW
Suite 315
Washington, D.C. 20009
(202) 483–2600

Florida Division, Inc.
1001 South MacDill Avenue
Tampa, Florida 33629
(813) 253–0541

Georgia Division, Inc.
46 Fifth Street, NE
Atlanta, Georgia 30308
(404) 892–0026

Hawaii/Pacific Division, Inc.
Community Services Center
  Bldg.
200 North Vineyard
  Boulevard
Honolulu, Hawaii 96817
(808) 531–1662

Idaho Division, Inc.
2676 Vista Avenue
P.O. Box 5386
Boise, Idaho 83705
(208) 343–4609

Illinois Division, Inc.
77 East Monroe
Chicago, Illinois 60603
(312) 641–6150

Indiana Division, Inc.
8730 Commerce Park Place
Indianapolis, Indiana 46268
(317) 872–4432

Iowa Division, Inc.
8364 Hickman Road, Suite D
Des Moines, Iowa 50322
(515) 253–0147

Kansas Division, Inc.
1315 SW Arrowhead Road
Topeka, Kansas 66604
(913) 273–4114

Kentucky Division, Inc.
701 West Muhammed Ali
  Blvd.

P.O. Box 1807
Louisville, Kentucky
  40217–1807
(502) 584–6782

Louisiana Division, Inc.
Fidelity Homestead Bldg.
837 Gravier Street
Suite 700
New Orleans, Louisiana
  70112–1509
(504) 523–2029

Maine Division, Inc.
52 Federal Street
Brunswick, Maine 04011
(207) 729–3339

Maryland Division, Inc.
8219 Town Center Drive
P.O. Box 82
White Marsh, Maryland
  21162–0082
(301) 529–7272

Massachusetts Division, Inc.
247 Commonwealth Avenue
Boston, Massachusetts 02116
(617) 267–2650

Michigan Division, Inc.
1205 East Saginaw Street
Lansing, Michigan 48906
(517) 371–2920

Minnesota Division, Inc.
3316 West 66th Street

Minneapolis, Minnesota
  55435
(612) 925–2772

Mississippi Division, Inc.
1380 Livingston Lane
Lakeover Office Park
Jackson, Mississippi 39213
(601) 362–8874

Missouri Division, Inc.
3322 American Avenue
Jefferson City, Missouri
  65102
(314) 893–4800

Montana Division, Inc.
313 N. 32nd Street
Suite #1
Billings, Montana 59101
(406) 252–7111

Nebraska Division, Inc.
8502 West Center Road
Omaha, Nebraska
  68124–5255
(402) 393–5800

Nevada Division, Inc.
1325 East Harmon
Las Vegas, Nevada 89119
(702) 798–6857

New Hampshire Division,
  Inc.
360 Route 101, Unit 501

Bedford, New Hampshire
  03102–6800
(603) 472–8899

New Jersey Division, Inc.
2600 Route 1, CNN 2201
North Brunswick, New Jersey
  08902
(201) 297–8000

New Mexico Division, Inc.
5800 Lomas Blvd., N.E.
Albuquerque, New Mexico
  87110
(505) 260–2105

New York State Division,
  Inc.
6725 Lyons Street
P.O. Box 7
East Syracuse, New York
  13057
(315) 437–7025

Long Island Division, Inc.
145 Pidgeon Hill Road
Huntington Station, New
  York 11746
(516) 385–9100

New York City Division, Inc.
19 West 56th Street
New York, New York 10019
(212) 586–8700

Queens Division, Inc.
112–25 Queens Boulevard

Forest Hills, New York
  11375
(718) 263–2224

Westchester Division, Inc.
30 Glenn St.
White Plains, New York
  10603
(914) 949–4800

North Carolina Division, Inc.
11 South Boylan Avenue
Suite 221
Raleigh, North Carolina
  27603
(919) 834–8463

North Dakota Division, Inc.
123 Roberts Street
P.O. Box 426
Fargo, North Dakota 58107
(701) 232–1385

Ohio Division, Inc.
5555 Frantz Road
Dublin, Ohio 43017
(614) 889–9565

Oklahoma Division, Inc.
300 United Founders Blvd.
Suite 136
Oklahoma City, Oklahoma
  73112
(405) 843–9888

Oregon Division, Inc.
0330 SW Curry Street

Portland, Oregon 97201
(503) 295–6422

Pennsylvania Division, Inc.
P.O. Box 897
Route 422 & Sipe Avenue
Hershey, Pennsylvania
  17033–0897
(717) 533–6144

Philadelphia Division, Inc.
1422 Chestnut Street
Philadelphia, Pennsylvania
  19102
(215) 665–2900

Puerto Rico Division, Inc.
Calle Alverio #577
Esquina Sargento Medina
Hato Rey, Puerto Rico 00918
(809) 764–2295

Rhode Island Division, Inc.
400 Main Street
Pawtucket, Rhode Island
  02860
(401) 722–8480

South Carolina Division, Inc.
128 Stonemark Lane
Columbia, South Carolina
  29210
(803) 750–1693

South Dakota Division, Inc.
4101 Carnegie Circle

Sioux Falls, South Dakota
  57106–2322
(605) 361–8277

Tennessee Division, Inc.
1315 Eighth Avenue South
Nashville, Tennessee 37203
(615) 255–1ACS

Texas Division, Inc.
2433 Ridgepoint Drive
Austin, Texas 78754
(512) 928–2262

Utah Division, Inc.
610 East South Temple
Salt Lake City, Utah 84102
(801) 322–0431

Vermont Division, Inc.
13 Loomis Street, Drawer C
P.O. Box 1452
Montpelier, Vermont
  05602–1452
(802) 223–2348

Virginia Division, Inc.
4240 Park Place Court
Glen Allen, Virginia 23060
(804) 270–0142/
  (800) ACS–2345

Washington Division, Inc.
2120 First Avenue North
Seattle, Washington
  98109–1140
(206) 283–1152

West Virginia Division, Inc.
2428 Kanawha Boulevard
East Charleston,
  West Virginia 25311
(304) 344–3611

Wisconsin Division, Inc.
615 North Sherman Avenue
Madison, Wisconsin 53704
(608) 249–0487

Wyoming Division, Inc.
2222 House Avenue
Cheyenne, Wyoming 82001
(307) 638–3331

Canadians can contact:

Canadian Cancer Society
77 Bloor Street, Suite 1702
Toronto, Ontario M5S3A1
(416) 961–7223

"I Can Cope," an eight-week hospital-based support and educational series, is one of the American Cancer Society's more popular programs. In classes and discussions, members of the hospital's treatment team provide information to patients and their relatives about cancer causes and side effects and counsel them about coping with the illness and its physical and emotional consequences. Contact your state's American Cancer Society division to find out if there is a hospital in your area that participates in the program.

United Ostomy Association

This organization, largely administered by persons who have ostomies themselves, provides information and rehabilitative support to help patients, who have recently had a colostomy or similar surgery, return to a normal life. Upon request and with the approval of the physician, volunteers will visit patients at the hospital or in their home. The association publishes a magazine and over 500 local chapters conduct monthly meetings. Contact the national headquarters to get the location of the chapter nearest you.

> United Ostomy Association
> 36 Executive Park, Suite 120
> Irvine, CA 92714
> (1)–(800) 826–0826

Crohn's and Colitis Foundation of America

Founded in 1967, CCFA (until recently called the National Foundation for Ileitis and Colitis) is the only nonprofit, voluntary health organization that actively funds research and education in inflammatory bowel disease. The foundation's primary goal is to raise funds for its nationwide biomedical research program to find the cause and cure for Crohn's disease and ulcerative colitis, but CCFA also conducts extensive campaigns to inform patients, physicians, and the public about the nature of these diseases and their complications. With over 20,000 members— health professionals as well as Crohn's and colitis patients— CCFA has 86 chapters and branches across the country. Members pay a $25 annual fee and receive the national newsletter and chapter bulletins, current research reports, and publication discounts. They also are able to participate in discount vitamin and prescription medicine programs, and are invited to attend chapter events and educational meetings.

National Headquarters
444 Park Avenue South
New York, New York
    10016-7374
    (1)–(800) 932–2423

Regional Offices

Northeast Regional Office
94 Church Street, Suite 203
New Brunswick, NJ
    08901-1226
(201) 214–0505

Mid-Atlantic Regional Office
3701 Old Court Road
    Suite 24
Baltimore, MD 21208-3901
(301) 486–9511

Midwest Regional Office
395 East Dundee Road
    Suite 450

Wheeling, IL 60090-7005
(708) 459–6342

South/Southwest Regional
    Office
One Davis Boulevard
    Suite 707
Tampa, FL 33606-3467
(813) 251–2191

Western Regional Office
9740 Washington Boulevard
Culver City, CA 90232-2722
(213) 559–8667

Information on Carcinogens

The following federal agencies provide free up-to-date information on specific products, food additives, and substances that have been suspected of causing cancer:

Consumer Products Safety Commission
Publication Request
Washington, DC 20207

Food and Drug Administration
Office for Consumer Communications
5600 Fishers Lane, Room 15B-32
Rockville, MD 20857
(301) 443–3170

Nutrition Information

The following organizations offer publications, some free of charge, featuring general nutrition information:

American Society for Clinical
  Nutrition
9650 Rockville Pike
Bethesda, MD 20814
(301) 530–7180

National Academy of
  Sciences
National Research Council
Food and Nutrition Board

2101 Constitution Avenue
  NW
Washington, DC 20418
(202) 334–1732

Human Nutrition
  Information Service
Nutrition Education and
  Research Branch
6505 Belcrest Road
Room 353

Hyattsville, MD 20776
(301) 436–5194

Nutrition Coordinating
  Committee

National Institutes of Health
Building 31, Room 4B-63
9000 Rockville Pike
Bethesda, MD 20892
(301) 496–9281

Glossary

Adenoma. A growth, usually benign, of tumor cells.

Anastomosis. Reconnection of the intestine after surgical resection of a diseased segment.

Antioncogene. A gene involved in controlling cellular growth; its absence or mutation can lead to unchecked cell proliferation. Also called a *tumor-suppressor gene*.

Ascending colon. Portion of the large intestine extending from the cecum up the right side of the abdomen toward the liver.

Benign. Noncancerous; not harmful to health.

Biopsy. Removal and examination of living tissue from the body.

Carcinogen. An environmental substance or agent that causes changes in the DNA, producing cancer or inciting its development.

Cecum. The first portion of the large intestine, a pouch on the lower right side of the abdomen connected to the ileum.

Chromosomes. Rod-shaped collection of genetic material in the nucleus of the cell, directing its action. Humans have 23 pairs of chromosomes in each normal cell.

Colectomy. Surgical excision of a section or all of the colon. A *hemicolectomy* involves the entire right or left side of the colon; a *subtotal colectomy* involves the whole colon except for the rectum.

Colonoscopy. Visual examination (using a colonoscope) of the entire inner surface of the colon.

Colostomy. Surgical formation of an opening *(stoma)* on the abdominal surface to allow the passage of body waste. A colostomy may be temporary, while the intestine heals after surgery, or permanent if the rectum has been resected.

Crohn's disease. Chronic inflammation of the intestinal tract, occurring most often in the last portion of the ileum.

Descending colon. Portion of the large intestine that turns downward from the transverse colon on the left side of the abdomen below the spleen.

Diverticula. Abnormal pockets, or outpouchings, in the bowel wall.

DNA (deoxyribonucleic acid). Genetic material within the nucleus of a cell, constructed of a double helix held together by hydrogen bonds, that transmits the hereditary pattern of the cell in humans and other cellular organisms.

Dysplasia. Abnormal, excessive accumulation of cells.

Endoscopy. Examination of a body cavity using an optical instrument.

Enema. Rectal injection of a liquid solution. Used to clear out the large bowel, or, in the case of a *barium enema,* to illuminate the intestine for X-ray examination.

Familial polyposis. Inherited condition causing the development of multiple polyps (hundreds or even thousands) along the lining throughout the large intestine. The condition usually appears by puberty, and, left untreated, almost invariably leads to cancer.

Fiber. Chemical substance that makes up plant cell walls. The term also commonly refers to the other indigestible parts of fruits and vegetables.

First-degree relative. Direct biological relatives of the same generation or one removed: biological parents, full siblings, and children.

Genes. Basic units of heredity, determining all inherited characteristics, situated in fixed locations within the chromosome.

Genome. The complete set of genes in an individual or organism.

Ileum. The last division of the small intestine; an 11-foot long section ending in the lower right side of the abdomen, where it connects to the cecum.

Immunotherapy. Treatment that uses the body's own defense mechanisms to prevent or delay the recurrence of cancer. Also called *biotherapy.*

Initiation. The first stage of cancer formation, when a carcinogen begins to alter healthy cells so that they start growing in an uncontrolled manner.

Irritable bowel syndrome. A group of intestinal symptoms (including abdominal pain and abnormal bowel functions) associated with stress and tension. Sometimes called "spastic colon."

Lipoma. A benign tumor, usually composed of fatty tissue.

Lymphatic system. The lymph nodes, bone marrow, spleen, and thymus gland. The system circulates nutrients throughout the body and produces and stores infection-fighting cells.

Lymphocytes. White blood cells formed in lymphatic tissue by the immune system.

Malignant. Cancerous; tending to become worse and threatening to cause death.

Metastasis. The spread of cancer from one part of the body to a secondary site.

Monoclonal antibody. A protein, produced by cloning mouse cells, that can neutralize or counteract the proliferation of a tumor by binding to it.

Oncogene. A gene whose activation is associated with the conversion of normal tumor cells into cancer cells.

Polyp. A small, usually harmless, mass of tissue that projects from the mucus membrane surface.

Polypectomy. Excision of a polyp.

Proctitis. Inflammation of the rectum.

Promotion. An early stage in cancer development, when agents that are not necessarily carcinogenic stimulate tumor formation.

Rectum. The final section of the large intestine, extending from the sigmoid colon to the anal canal.

Resection. Surgical removal of part or all of an organ.

Sigmoid colon. The s-shaped portion of the large bowel at the lower end of the descending colon.

Sigmoidoscopy. Visual examination (using a rigid or flexible sigmoidoscope) of the lower portion of the large intestine; also called *proctosigmoidoscopy* or *proctoscopy*.

Sporadic cancer. Malignancy that occurs in an apparently random or isolated manner, neither related to nor influenced by a clearly defined genetic disorder.

Stoma. A small, artificial opening in the abdominal wall created during intestinal surgery, through which a portion of the bowel is attached to allow the elimination of body waste.

Transverse colon. The portion of the large bowel under the stomach extending right to left across the abdomen, from the ascending colon to the descending colon.

Ulcerative colitis. Chronic ulceration and inflammation involving part of or the entire colon and rectum.

Index